Healthy Cooking

Fat Loss with Clean Eating

Karen Parker and Irene Carter

Table of Contents

CHAPTER 7: BELLY FLATTENING DRINK, SNACK AND DESSERT RECIPES

CHAPTER 8: YOUR 7 DAY BELLY FAT DIET MEAL PLAN

Introduction

Going on a diet is tough enough, if you are going on a diet because you want to practice better nutrition or if you are wanting to lose weight and fat. The reason why does not matter. Going on a low calorie diet can be difficult because you may feel hungry from barely eating. Going on a low carb diet may make you feel the cravings for carbs strongly. This dieting cookbook contains recipes from two different diet plans, the Eating Clean diet and the Belly Fat diet. All of the recipes are home cooking and tastes great. You will not lack for flavor, nor will you feel hungry from the recipes in this book, but you will achieve your goal of eating healthier and losing fat and weight.

There is no right or wrong way to use this cookbook. It does have two different diet plans, so you have three ways you can use this book. You can specifically use the eating clean diet if you wish to put nothing but clean nutritious foods in your body to be healthier. You can go on the belly fat diet, which will help you to lose weight and belly fat. Or you can choose from both diets. Really, the eating clean diet will help you to lose weight just fine too. You could go on the belly fat diet and lose the weight you wish to lose, and then switch to the eating clean diet for weight maintenance. If you choose to use the recipes in the whole book, you will have several weeks' worth of meal plans without repeating a meal. This is a delicious way to become healthy and lose weight.

Changing the dieting lifestyle can take a couple of weeks to get accustomed to doing. You will want to let go of the junk foods you are consuming, like processed flours and sugars, foods with saturated fats, convenient foods, and fast foods. These foods are not considered "clean eating" nor will they help you to lose belly fat. In fact, they will help you to gain belly fat, just the opposite of what you hope to achieve. Junk foods have a way of grabbing hold of our appetites though and this is why so many struggle with nutrition. They crave the junk foods over the nutritious foods. The good news is that the recipes in this book are both healthy and tasty, so you will not feel too deprived here. If you have a severe junk food addiction, you may wish to wean off that before jumping into the dieting fully.

In order to make the diets in this book a bigger success takes some time to wean off of the junk foods first. It takes the body about three weeks to break and addiction. You will be so glad you did because you do not want to be craving the junk while you are eating the healthy foods. Of course, the recipes in this book are the best of home cooking and they taste as good too, so it will help. To wean successfully from junk replace a junk snack or meal every three days with the meals and recipes in this book. By three weeks, you should have successfully weaned from the junk food. You will feel a lot better too and you will have more energy.

Once you wean from the junk food habits, you will be ready to focus on your dieting health. Other simple things you can do now can help make your change in lifestyle successful. You want to be healthier you must work to let go of other bad habits you may have such as smoking, excessive alcohol consumption, or even taking recreational drugs. Letting go of these bad habits will add healthy years to your life. But there are still more things you can do to insure you are at your healthiest.

Make drinking water a big part of your day. The body needs a lot of water in order to stay hydrated. Take your weight in pounds and divide by 2. If you weight 200 lbs. - divide it by 2 you have 100. A person weighing 200 pounds needs 100 ounces of water a day. That is 12 cups of water a day. Now if you do an exercise workout you need to add another 12 ounces to replace the water you will lose during the workout. Drinking water helps the body to clean itself from the inside out. Drinking water helps the body to assimilate the food you eat and if you are eating healthy foods, your body is able to pull out the nutrients it needs.

Make sure you get plenty of rest daily. If you are unable to get 6 to 8 hours of sleep per night, you will need to make up for it. Taking a quick catnap will help to recharge the body. It only takes about 20 minutes of rest to rejuvenate. Set an alarm and do not sleep longer. If you are unable to rest for 20 uninterrupted minutes at a time, then take shorter rest periods throughout the day. Ideally, you will want to rest your eyes and mind for 5 to 10 minutes throughout the day. Make it your goal though to get more sleep at night if you are going under 6 hours. Try to rearrange your schedule and better prioritize your time.

Add in some exercise to help make the dieting better. Exercise is healthy for the body. You only need to do it every other day and only for a half an hour at a time in order to be effective. The diets work better with a body that is physically active too. Always clear any diet changes and exercise routines with your health care provider before starting a new diet program. The recipes within this book contain nutritious foods, but your health care provider will be able to tell you if they are right for you.

Section 1: Eating Clean Diet

What is the eating clean diet?

The eating clean diet also called, clean eating diet or the eat clean diet, is a very simple and basic diet. It is the absence of anything chemical including processed flours and sugars, chemicals and preservatives, artificial dyes and flavors. It is food in its most natural state, the way it comes off the vine or plant or tree. It is food that you pick up at the produce section or from the freezer. You can find this food in the canned goods as well. Clean food diet is exactly what it sounds like.

Why Eat Clean Foods?

Eating foods on this diet puts you back to as close to nature as possible eating foods in their natural state without any processing or unnecessary ingredients. The body is able to assimilate foods better. It acts as a cleanse at first helping the body to detoxify from all the additives and preservatives. Natural foods help to keep the digestive system clean by acting as a natural scrubber as it goes through the tract.

Can you lose weight on this diet?

That is a big yes. Why? Because by not eating junk food the body has a chance to use all the nutrients that comes from clean foods to help boost the metabolism. This means that it digests the foods at the perfect time, pulling all the necessary nutrients out. Because there are no bad fats or sugars in natural foods the body does not hang on to them like it does when you consumer junk food. Because natural foods help the body to speed up the metabolism, you have more energy and when you have more energy you feel like getting up and moving around. Developing and maintaining a good exercise routine is vital in weight loss and very possible when consuming clean foods because you will have that extra energy.

Is the clean food diet healthy?

Yes. Consuming clean foods helps to boost the immune system. How? The best way to receive all the nutrients you need (nutrients as in vitamins, minerals, complex carbohydrates and more) is through the foods you eat. If you are eating whole healthy foods then your body is receiving all the nutrients it needs in order to keep you healthy.

The clean diet includes all the "super foods" like quinoa,

spinach, and fruits and vegetables. These foods are high in nutrients and in particular in anti-oxidants. Anti-oxidants are vitamins and minerals that help to attack and get rid of free radicals in the body. Free radicals are substances that cause horrible diseases like cancer, heart disease and other debilitating diseases. If the body is able to fight free radicals it means the immune system is strong and healthy. And simply eating clean foods makes this happen.

Tips to make the eating clean diet work.

When you go grocery shopping of course you want to focus on all foods that are not labeled as "convenient food" or junk food. You will want to shop in the produce section (or your local farmer's market if available), the frozen foods section, and for canned goods.

Read labels. That is the only way you can be 100% sure you are purchasing truly clean foods. Read labels especially if you are purchasing prepackaged foods. Be very careful here. Even canned fruits and vegetables can contain unnecessary ingredients.

A general rule of thumb is if the ingredients are unrecognizable words, words with a lot of letters, words you cannot pronounce, they are probably preservatives and artificial colors and artificial flavors. Do not buy anything like this. Even if the package says it is all natural, always read the ingredients list. You can find some prepackaged foods that are all natural. But always read the labels.

If you cannot find certain natural foods at your regular grocery, you can always look at health food stores or whole food stores and find them. If all else fails seek out recipes to make your own from wholesome ingredients.

The recipes in this book calls for certain foods you can purchase and may consider prepackaged. Bread is one ingredient called for in several recipes. It is recommended to find a bread that has on the label that it contains no trans fats and no preservatives. Read the ingredients. You can find whole grain breads that are all natural.

Cooking spray is very handy to have. You can find sprays that are made from canola oil or olive oil. Avoid the ones that are "butter flavored" as they may contain artificial flavorings.

Yogurt is another food called for in some of the ingredients. You can find all natural plain yogurts in most grocery stores and certainly in whole foods or health food stores. Vanilla extract is another ingredient in some of the recipes. Be sure to get the 100% pure vanilla extract and not the imitation, which is full of chemicals.

Soy sauce comes in all natural forms, so read the labels and purchase the ones that contains all wholesome ingredients and avoid the others. Salsa is another ingredient you can purchase already made, and it is fairly easy to find jars of all natural salsas. If you cannot find them on the shelves, look in the produce section or the deli for store made, which are normally all natural. If you cannot find any that is all natural, salsa is easy to make. There are a few recipes in this book for some.

Vegetable stock is another ingredient (as well as chicken and sometimes you can use beef stock). Be careful when purchasing these, read the labels. Some are 100% all natural and organic and these are the best ones to purchase. You can also make your own when cooking vegetables, chicken, and beef.

Tomato sauces and pastes are called for in some of the ingredients. You can find all natural cans of these on most grocery shelves, just read the labels. If you cannot find them, make your own, it is not that hard.

Just Start!

Knowing what you can and cannot eat on this diet is easy, all you have to do is go grocery shopping and avoid the junk foods and the processed foods and you will do well. The good news is you do not have to order special meals, or join a club, or spend a lot of extra money on specialty diet foods to go on this diet. You just go shopping and buy whole healthy foods and you are on your way to healthy eating. Give your body a chance to be healthier and to feel better by eating the clean diet foods. This is a change in lifestyle and a change you will want to keep. Losing weight will come naturally if you are overweight. All you have to do is stay on the diet and not eat junk food. It helps to add exercise with it, because exercising will help to lose weight faster.

Lastly, always check with your health care provider before starting any new diet or exercise routine and make sure the foods you will be eating are good foods for you.

Disclaimer: the recipes within this book are tried and true recipes that have been around for years in some form or another. Enjoy trying the recipes, feel free to adjust to your own tastes, and needs.

5 Day Sample Meal Plan

Below is a sample meal plan that covers 5 days. For snacks and desserts it is good to include whole nuts and fruits. With the main dishes, include a green salad and steamed vegetables.

Day 1

Breakfast - Baked Oatmeal
Snack - Banana
Lunch - Spicy Black Beans and Quinoa
Snack - Sweet and Spicy Mango Salsa with whole grain chips
Supper - Baked Italian Crusted Cod
Dessert - Baked Cinnamon Apple Toast

Day 2

Breakfast - Turkey Sausage Casserole
Snack - Guacamole with whole grain chips
Lunch - Tuna Salad
Snack - Walnuts
Supper - Basic Spaghetti Sauce over spaghetti squash
Dessert - Peanut Butter Balls

Day 3

Breakfast - Strawberry Banana Oat Smoothie

Snack - Dried apricots

Lunch - Chicken Chili

Snack - Hummus Dip

Supper - Turkey Meatloaf with Spicy Roasted Baked Potatoes

Dessert - Cinnamon Popcorn

Day 4

Breakfast - Breakfast Fruit Salad Snack - Deviled Eggs

Lunch - Asparagus Mushroom Roast

Snack - Apple

Supper - Honey Mustard Chicken with Oven Roasted Vegetables

Dessert - Banana Oat Cookies

Day 5

Breakfast - Raisin Quinoa Pudding

Snack - Banana

Lunch - Tangy Vegetable Salad

Snack - Almonds

Supper - Orange Lime Shrimp with Cabbage Summer Casserole

Dessert - Fruit Salad with Yogurt Dressing (from the

breakfast recipes)

Eating Clean Diet Recipes

Breakfast Recipes

Apple Muffins

Here is a gluten free recipe using rice flour in a delicious muffin. Makes 6 muffins.

What You'll Need:

2 apples (Gala, peeled, cored, fine diced)
1 egg
1 cup of flour (white rice)
2/3 cup of yogurt (plain)
1/4 cup of oats (steel cut)
1/4 cup of cranberry juice
1 1/2 tablespoons of butter (melted)
1 tablespoon of flax seed
1 teaspoon of baking soda
1 teaspoon of cinnamon (ground)
1/2 teaspoon of nutmeg (ground)
1/2 teaspoon of arrowroot powder

How to Make It:

Prep: Preheat the oven to 350 degrees Fahrenheit. Spray a large 6 cup muffin pan with cooking spray. In a bowl mix the dry ingredients of 1 cup of flour (white rice), 1/4 cup of oats (steel cut), 1 tablespoon of flax seed, 1 teaspoon of baking soda, 1 teaspoon of cinnamon (ground), 1/2 teaspoon of nutmeg (ground), and the 1/2 teaspoon of arrowroot powder. In a separate bowl add the egg and beat with a whisk, then add the 2/3 cup of yogurt (plain), 1/4 cup of cranberry juice, and 1 1/2 tablespoons of butter (melted) and stir. Gradually add the dry ingredients and stir until just combined. Stir in the 2 apples (Gala, peeled, cored, fine diced). Pour evenly into the 6 large muffin cups. Bake until the muffins are golden brown, when a toothpick inserted in the middle of a muffin emerges clean, about half an hour. Cool for a couple of minutes and serve.

Baked Oatmeal

This delicious bowl of oatmeal has blueberries, applesauce, and cinnamon. Makes 8 servings.

What You'll Need:

3 cups of oats (rolled)
2 eggs
1 cups of blueberries (frozen)
1 cups of milk
1/2 cup of applesauce
1/2 cup of honey
1/8 cup of flax seed meal
1 1/2 tablespoons of wheat germ
1/2 tablespoon of baking powder
1/2 tablespoon of cinnamon (ground)
1 teaspoons of vanilla extract
1/4 teaspoons of salt
Butter
Milk

How to Make It:

Prep: Preheat the oven to 350 degrees Fahrenheit.

Mix the 3 cups of oats (rolled), 2 beaten eggs, 1 cups of

blueberries (frozen), 1 cups of milk, 1/2 cup of applesauce, 1/2 cup of honey, 1/8 cup of flax seed meal, 1 1/2 tablespoons of wheat germ, 1/2 tablespoon of baking powder, 1/2 tablespoon of cinnamon (ground), 1 teaspoons of vanilla extract, and 1/4 teaspoons of salt in a large bowl. Pour into a 9x9 inch baking dish or casserole dish. Bake for half an hour. Add extra butter and milk if desired when serving.

Blended Fruit Breakfast

This is a delicious and refreshing yet filling breakfast. Makes 2 servings.

What You'll Need:

6 apricots (dried, chopped)
1 cup of yogurt (plain)
1/2 cup of milk
1/2 cup of oats (rolled)
1/4 cup of oat bran
2 tablespoons of raisins
2 teaspoons of walnuts (chopped)
Ground cinnamon

How to Make It:

The night before: Combine the 6 apricots (dried, chopped), 1 cup of yogurt (plain), 1/2 cup of oats (rolled), 1/4 cup of oat bran, 2 tablespoons of raisins, and dashes of ground cinnamon. Cover and set in refrigerator. Next morning, divide between 2 bowls, pour 1/4 cup of milk and sprinkle 1 teaspoon of chopped walnuts over the top, serve.

Breakfast Fruit Salad

This is a refreshing breakfast, perfect for a hot summer morning, or as an anytime snack. Makes 10 servings.

What You'll Need:

3 kiwis (peeled, sliced)
3 bananas (peeled, sliced, ripe)
2 oranges (peeled, sectioned)
2 cups of pineapple (cubed)
2 cups of strawberries (hulled, sliced)
2 cups of blueberries
1 cup of grapes (seedless)
2/3 cups of orange juice
1/3 cup of lemon juice
1/3 cup of honey
1 teaspoon of vanilla extract
1/2 teaspoon of lemon zest
1/2 teaspoon of orange zest

How to Make It:

Pour the 2/3 cups of orange juice, 1/3 cup of honey, 1/3 cup of lemon juice, 1/2 teaspoon of lemon zest, and the 1/2 teaspoon of orange zest into a saucepan, stir and turn heat to medium high to bring to a boil. Turn to medium low, stir and cook for an additional 5 minutes. Stir in the 1 teaspoon of vanilla extract and set aside. In a large serving bowl (a large salad bowl works well) combine the 3 kiwis (peeled, sliced), 3 bananas (peeled, sliced, ripe), 2 oranges (peeled, sectioned), 2 cups of pineapple (cubed), 2 cups of strawberries (hulled, sliced), 2 cups of blueberries, and the 1 cup of grapes (seedless). Drizzle the cooked fruit juice over the top and toss. Place in the refrigerator for about 3 1/2 hours to chill before serving.

Coconut Oatmeal

Nothing quite satisfies hunger like a nice hot bowl of oatmeal first thing in the morning. Makes 6 servings.

What You'll Need:

3 1/2 cups of milk
2 cups of oats (rolled)
1 cup of yogurt (plain)
1/3 cup of raisins
1/3 cup of cranberries (dried)
1/3 cup of coconut (flaked)
1/3 cup of walnuts (chopped)
1/4 cup of maple syrup (pure)
3 tablespoons of honey
1/4 teaspoon of salt

How to Make It:

Add the 3 1/2 cups of milk and the 1/4 teaspoon of salt to a saucepan over high heat and carefully bring to a boil, watching and stirring constantly. Add the 2 cups of oats (rolled), 1/3 cup of raisins, 1/3 cup of cranberries (dried), and the 1/4 cup of maple syrup (pure), bring the mixture to a second boil, stirring constantly. Turn the heat down to medium and cook for another 5 minutes.

Add the 1/3 cup of coconut (flaked) and the 1/3 cup of walnuts (chopped), stir and cut the heat. Spoon into 6 bowls and divide the cup of plain yogurt and the 3 tablespoons of honey evenly among the bowls. Serve and enjoy.

French Toast

Everyone loves a batch of French toast for breakfast, a tasty sweet way to start the day. Makes 6 servings.

What You'll Need:

6 slices of whole grain bread
6 pats of butter
4 eggs
2/3 cup of milk
1 teaspoon of vanilla extract
1/2 teaspoon of cinnamon (ground)
Pure maple syrup

How to Make It:

Crack the 4 eggs into a shallow bowl and beat with a whisk. Add the 2/3 cup of milk, teaspoon of vanilla extract and the 1/2 teaspoon of ground cinnamon and stir to combine. Heat a skillet or griddle to medium high heat, spray with cooking spray. Dip each slice of bread in the egg mixture, coating all of it. Place on the hot skillet or griddle and cook until it turns a golden brown on the bottom, the flip and do the same. Repeat with each slice. Place a pat of butter on the hot toast. Drizzle with pure maple syrup and enjoy.

Fruit Salad with Yogurt Dressing

This is a refreshing breakfast with fresh fruit and a tangy yet sweet yogurt dressing. Makes 8 servings.

What You'll Need:

2 kiwis (peeled, chopped)
1 can of pineapples (crushed, 15 oz., in natural juices)
2 cups of yogurt (plain)
1 cup of grapes (red)
1 cup of strawberries (hulled, chopped)
1 cup of blueberries
1 cup of Granny Smith apples (cored, chopped)
1 cup of Fuji apples (cored, chopped)
2 tablespoons of lemon juice
2 tablespoons of honey

How to Make It:

Toss and combine the 2 kiwis (peeled, chopped), 1 can of pineapples (crushed, 15 oz., in natural juices), 1 cup of grapes (red), 1 cup of strawberries (hulled, chopped), 1 cup of blueberries, 1 cup of Granny Smith apples (cored, chopped), and the 1 cup of Fuji apples (cored, chopped) in a large bowl. In a small bowl add the 2 cups of plain yogurt, 2 tablespoons of lemon juice and 2 tablespoons of honey and stir with a whisk. Pour over the fruit and toss to coat.   Serve and enjoy or store in the refrigerator.

Raisin Quinoa Pudding

This is a delightful breakfast with apple juice, raisins, and the super food quinoa. Makes 6 servings.

What You'll Need:

2 cups of water
2 cups of apple juice
1 cup of raisins
1 cup of quinoa
2 tablespoons of lemon juice
1 teaspoon of cinnamon (ground)
2 teaspoons of vanilla extract
Salt (if desired)

How to Make It:

Rinse the cup of quinoa in cheesecloth, squeezing out the excess. Add the quinoa to a saucepan and put the 2 cups of water over it. Turn to high heat and bring to a boil. Cover the saucepan and turn to low to simmer for about 15 minutes, until all the water is absorbed. Add the 2 cups of apple juice, 1 cup of raisins, 2 tablespoons of lemon juice, and 1 teaspoon of cinnamon (ground). Stir in salt if desired. Cook for 15 minutes on low, with lid on. Add the 2 teaspoons of vanilla extract at the last stir and serve.

Strawberry, Banana, Oat Smoothie

Sometimes you can simply drink your breakfast such as this delicious fruit smoothie. Makes 2 servings.

What You'll Need:

1 banana (peeled, chunked, frozen)
1 1/4 cup of strawberries (frozen)
1 cup of milk
1/2 cup of oats (rolled)
1/4 cup of ice
2 teaspoons of honey
1/2 teaspoon of vanilla extract

How to Make It:

Add the 1 banana (peeled, chunked, frozen), 1 1/4 cup of strawberries (frozen), 1 cup of milk, 1/2 cup of oats (rolled), 1/4 cup of ice, 2 teaspoons of honey, and the 1/2 teaspoon of vanilla extract into a blender or food processor and blend until smooth. Pour in a glass and enjoy.

Toasted PB and B

This is a toasted whole grain bread with natural peanut butter and bananas. Kids will love this breakfast. Makes 2 servings.

What You'll Need:

4 slices of whole grain bread
2 bananas
1/4 cup of peanut butter (natural creamy)
4 pats of butter

How to Make It:

Spread 1/8 cup of natural creamy peanut butter onto 2 slices of the whole grain bread. Peel and slice a banana on top of each peanut butter spread bread. Place another slice of whole grain bread on top the bananas. Add a pat of butter to a non-stick skillet over medium high heat and toast one side of one of the sandwiches. Repeat until both sides of each sandwich is toasted. Serve.

Turkey Sausage Casserole

This delicious casserole is wholesome and filling. Makes 8 servings.

What You'll Need:

1 pound of turkey sausage
6 slices of whole grain bread (toasted, cubed)
4 eggs
2 cups of milk
2 cups of cheddar cheese (mild, shredded)
1 teaspoon of mustard powder
Salt and pepper
Canola oil

How to Make It:

Prep: Preheat the oven to 350 degrees Fahrenheit. Spray a 9x13 inch baking dish with cooking spray.

Add a touch of canola oil to a skillet, then crumble and brown the pound of turkey sausage. Meanwhile, in a bowl, crack the 4 eggs and beat with a whisk. Combine with the 2 cups of milk, 1 teaspoon of mustard powder, and dashes of salt and pepper. Stir in the cooked turkey sausage, 6 slices of whole grain bread (toasted, cubed), and the 2 cups of cheddar cheese (mild, shredded). Pour into the prepared 9x13 inch baking dish and cover with foil and bake for 45 minutes. Turn the oven down to 325 degrees Fahrenheit, remove the foil cover, and bake for another half an hour, making sure the eggs are cooked. Let sit for 5 minutes before serving.

Vegetables Frittata

This is a delicious breakfast made with whole vegetables and fresh eggs. Makes 8 servings.

What You'll Need:

6 eggs
4 slices of whole grain bread (cubed)
2 packages of cream cheese (8 oz., diced, room temperature)
2 cups of cheddar cheese (sharp, shredded)
1 1/2 cups of zucchini (chopped)
1 1/2 cups of mushrooms (fresh chopped)
3/4 cup of onion (chopped)
3/4 cup of bell pepper (green chopped)
1/4 cup of half-and-half cream
3 tablespoons of canola oil
1/2 teaspoon of garlic (minced)
Salt and pepper

How to Make It:

Prep: Preheat the oven to 350 degrees Fahrenheit. Spray a 9x13 inch baking dish with cooking spray.

Pour the 3 tablespoons of canola oil into a skillet and

heat to medium high. Stir in the 1 1/2 cups of zucchini (chopped), 1 1/2 cups of mushrooms (fresh chopped), 3/4 cup of onion (chopped), 3/4 cup of bell pepper (green chopped), and the 1/2 teaspoon of garlic (minced) and sauté. Take off heat. In a bowl, crack the 6 eggs and beat with a whisk. Stir in the 1/4 cup of half-and-half cream. Then add the 4 slices of cubed whole grain bread, 2 8 oz. packages of diced cream cheese, 2 cups of cheddar cheese (sharp, shredded), and the cooked vegetables. Sprinkle dashes of salt and pepper and combine. Pour into the prepared 9x13 inch baking dish. Bake until the eggs set in the center, about 60 minutes. Allow to stand outside the oven for about 5 minutes before serving.

Whole Grain Pancakes

Drizzle your favorite pancake topping over these healthy whole grain pancakes for a delicious hot breakfast. Pure maple syrup recommended. Makes 4 servings.

What You'll Need:

2 eggs
2 cups of buttermilk
1 1/2 cups of flour (whole wheat pastry)
1/2 cup of wheat germ
1/4 cup of canola oil
2 teaspoons of baking soda
1/2 teaspoon of salt

How to Make It:

Mix the 1 1/2 cups of flour (whole wheat pastry), 1/2 cup of wheat germ, 1/2 teaspoons of baking soda, and 1/2 teaspoon of salt together. In a separate bowl, beat the 2 eggs with a whisk, then combine with the 2 cups of buttermilk, and 1/4 cup of canola oil. Add the dry ingredients and stir. Spray a griddle or large skillet with cooking spray and heat to medium high. Ladle a spoon of batter and cook until the edges dry and the center turns bubbly. Flip, repeat unto all the pancakes are made.

Eating Clean Diet Appetizers, Snacks, and Dessert Recipes

Baked Cinnamon Apple Toast

This is a quick and delicious snack, perfect for after school or as an impromptu dessert. Makes 4 servings.

What You'll Need:

1 apple (large, cored, sliced thin)
4 slices of whole grain bread
1 tablespoon of butter (room temperature, divided)
1 tablespoon of cinnamon (ground)
Honey

How to Make It:

Prep: Preheat the oven on broil (high).

Spread 1/4 tablespoon of butter onto one side of each slice of whole grain bread.   Lay the bread on a baking sheet, butter side facing up. Evenly disperse the apple slices on top of each slice of bread. Sprinkle a few dashes of cinnamon on top of the apples. Drizzle a little honey on top of the cinnamon and apples. Place under the broiler until the edges of the bread turns to toast, a couple of minutes.

Banana Oat Cookies

These cookies are delicious with a nice cold glass of milk. Makes 36 cookies.

What You'll Need:

2 cups of bananas (ripe, chopped)
2 cups of oats (rolled)
1 cup of dates (pitted, chopped)
1/3 cup of canola oil
1 teaspoon of vanilla extract

How to Make It:

Prep: Preheat the oven to 350 degrees Fahrenheit.

Place the 2 cups of chopped bananas in a large bowl and mash with a potato masher. Add the 2 cups of oats (rolled), 1 cup of dates (pitted, chopped), 1/3 cup of canola oil, and 1 teaspoon of vanilla extract and mix. Set aside for about 15 minutes, and then drop by the spoonful's onto a baking sheet. Bake until cookies turn a golden brown about 20 minutes. Cool a few minutes on a wire rack before serving.

Cinnamon Popcorn

Healthy and wholesome, this snack will satisfy those in between meal hunger pangs. Makes 6 servings.

What You'll Need:

3/4 cup of popcorn kernels
3 tablespoons of olive oil
2 tablespoons of honey
Salt
Cinnamon (ground)

How to Make It:

Using a large pot with a lid, heat the 3 tablespoons of olive oil on high heat for 2 minutes. Pour in the 3/4 cup of popcorn kernels and replace the lid. Move the pot over the heat to prevent burning, shaking especially when the corn is popping. Pull from heat when the popping slows.   Pour popped corn into a large bowl. Toss with the 2 tablespoons of honey, a couple dashes of salt and a dash or two of ground cinnamon.

Deviled Eggs

A classic recipe that always tastes great. Makes a dozen deviled eggs.

What You'll Need:

6 eggs
1 1/2 tablespoon of prepared mustard
1 1/2 tablespoon of mayonnaise
3/4 teaspoon of garlic salt
3/4 teaspoon of onion powder
Paprika
Water

How to Make It:

Put the 6 eggs into a medium saucepan and cover completely with cold water. Place saucepan on high heat and bring to a rapid boil for 10 minutes. Remove pan from heat and set on a cool burner for 5 minutes. Put pan in the sink and run cold water over the eggs. Let eggs sit in the cool water for a few minutes to cool. Remove the shells from the eggs and cut in half lengthwise. Carefully remove the yolks and place in a bowl. Add the 1 1/2 tablespoon of prepared mustard, 1 1/2 tablespoon of mayonnaise, 3/4 teaspoon of garlic salt, and 3/4 teaspoon of onion powder and mix well, incorporating the egg yolks into a creamy mixture. Spoon the egg yolk mixture back into the egg whites until it is all gone. Sprinkle with paprika. Store in the refrigerator for an hour before serving.

Guacamole

This is a great dip, great with Mexican dishes, and makes for wonderful snacks or appetizers. Makes 4 servings.

What You'll Need:

3 avocados (peeled, pitted, chopped)
1/4 cup of onions (diced)
3 tablespoons of cilantro (fresh chopped)
2 tablespoons of lime juice
1 teaspoon of garlic (minced)
Salt
Cayenne pepper

How to Make It:

Place the 3 avocados (peeled, pitted, chopped) in a blender or food processor and blend until smooth. Add in the 2 tablespoons of lime juice and several dashes of salt. Transfer to a bowl and combine with the 1/4 cup of onions (diced), 3 tablespoons of cilantro (fresh chopped) 1 teaspoon of garlic (minced), and a dash or two of the cayenne pepper. Refrigerate for half an hour before serving.

Hummus Dip

Enjoy a nutritious snack with pita chips or whole grain crackers. Makes 4 servings.

What You'll Need:

1 can of garbanzo beans (15 oz., drained but keep the liquid)
1 tablespoon of olive oil
2 teaspoons of cumin (ground)
1/2 teaspoon of garlic (minced)
Salt

How to Make It:

Add the 1 can of drained garbanzo beans, 1 tablespoon of olive oil, 2 teaspoons of cumin (ground), 1/2 teaspoon of garlic (minced), and dashes of salt into a food processor or blender and combine until smooth. Add the extra can liquid if needed.

Peanut Butter Balls

A delicious treat that both kids and adults love. If you are inclined, add a few semi-sweet chocolate chips to the mix. Makes 2 dozen.

What You'll Need:

1/2 cup of peanut butter (natural creamy)
1/3 cup of oats (rolled)
1/4 cup of apple juice (from the frozen can of concentrate, thawed)
1/4 cup of coconut (flakes)
1/4 cup of powdered milk
1/4 cup of wheat germ
1/2 teaspoon of cinnamon (ground)
Peanuts (finely chopped)

How to Make Them:

In a large bowl combine 1/2 cup of peanut butter (natural crunchy), 1/3 cup of oats (rolled), 1/4 cup of apple juice (from the frozen can of concentrate, thawed), 1/4 cup of coconut (flakes), 1/4 cup of powdered milk, 1/4 cup of wheat germ, and 1/2 teaspoon of cinnamon (ground). Roll into 2 dozen balls, then roll through the fine chopped peanuts.) Place in a container to store in the refrigerator.

Sweet and Spicy Mango Salsa

This is a different twist with a salsa, fruity yet hot and spicy. Makes 5 cups.

What You'll Need:

2 cups of Roma tomatoes (diced)
1 1/2 cups of mango (dried)
1/2 cup of cilantro (fresh chopped)
1/2 cup of onion (diced)
2 tablespoons of lime juice
1 tablespoon of apple cider vinegar
1 tablespoon of honey
1 teaspoon of garlic (minced)
Salt and pepper

How to Make It:

Combine the 2 cups of Roma tomatoes (diced), 1 1/2 cups of mango (dried), 1/2 cup of cilantro (fresh chopped), 1/2 cup of onion (diced), 2 tablespoons of lime juice, 1 tablespoon of apple cider vinegar, 1 tablespoon of honey, 1 teaspoon of garlic (minced), and dashes of salt and pepper in a large bowl. Cover and refrigerate for 60 minutes.

Eating Clean Diet Side Dish Recipes

Asparagus Mushroom Roast

You have a hit when you combine delicious asparagus with tasty mushrooms. Makes 6 servings.

What You'll Need:

.5 pound of mushrooms (fresh, quartered)
1 bunch of asparagus (trimmed)
2 sprigs of rosemary (minced)
2 teaspoons of olive oil
Salt and pepper

How to Make It:

Prep: Preheat oven to 450 degrees Fahrenheit. Line a baking sheet with foil and spray it with cooking spray.

Toss together the .5 pound of mushrooms (fresh, quartered), 1 bunch of asparagus (trimmed), 2 sprigs of rosemary (minced), 2 teaspoons of olive oil, and dashes of salt and pepper.   Spread on the prepared baking sheet and bake for 15 minutes, until the asparagus and mushrooms are tender.

Authentic Pico de Gallo

When eating south-of-the-border cuisine you need a delicious side dish of pico de gallo. Makes 4 servings.

What You'll Need:

2 sprigs of cilantro (chopped fine)
1 scallion (chopped fine)
1 tomato (diced)
1/2 jalapeno pepper (seeded, chopped)
1/2 cup of onions (chopped)
1/2 teaspoon of garlic (powder)
Salt and pepper

How to Make It:

Combine the 2 sprigs of cilantro (chopped fine), 1 scallion (chopped fine), 1 tomato (diced), 1/2 jalapeno pepper (seeded, chopped), 1/2 cup of onions (chopped), 1/2 teaspoon of garlic (powder), and dashes of salt and pepper in a bowl. Set in the refrigerator for half an hour at least before serving.

Beans and Peppers

This is a tasty dish made with great northern beans and banana peppers. Makes 4 servings.

What You'll Need:

1 can of great northern beans (drained)
2 banana peppers (chopped)
1/4 cup of onion (chopped)
1 teaspoon of olive oil
Oregano
Cayenne pepper
Salt and pepper

How to Make It:

Add the teaspoon of olive oil to a skillet heated to medium. Add the 2 banana peppers (chopped) and the 1/4 cup of onion (chopped) and sauté. Stir in the 1 can of great northern beans (drained), and dashes of oregano, cayenne pepper, salt and pepper. Keep on heat until heated through.

Cabbage Summer Casserole

This is a delightful dish with zucchini, squash and cabbage, you cannot go wrong with this. Makes 4 servings.

What You'll Need:

1 zucchini (sliced)
1 squash (yellow, sliced)
4 cups of cabbage (sliced)
2 cups of chicken stock
3/4 cup of onions (chopped)
Salt and pepper

How to Make It:

Combine the 1 zucchini (sliced), 1 squash (yellow, sliced), 4 cups of cabbage (sliced), 2 cups of chicken stock, 3/4 cup of onions (chopped), and dashes of salt and pepper in a large sauce pan and turn heat to high. Bring liquid to a boil, reduce heat to medium and continue cooking for 30 minutes.

Cauliflower and Greens

This is a delicious side dish made of cauliflower and kale with a refreshing lemon dressing. Makes 4 servings.

What You'll Need:

1 head of cauliflower (chopped bite-sized chunks)
1 bunch of kale (chopped)
4 cups of water
3 tablespoons of currants (dried)
2 tablespoons of olive oil (extra virgin)
1 tablespoon of Dijon mustard
1 tablespoon of lemon juice
2 teaspoons of lemon zest
Salt and pepper

How to Make It:

Combine the 1 tablespoon of Dijon mustard, 1 tablespoon of lemon juice, and the 2 teaspoons of lemon zest using a whisk. Add the 2 tablespoons of olive oil (extra virgin), whisk well. Stir in the 3 tablespoons of currants (dried).

Meanwhile, add the 4 cups of water to a steamer pot and turn to high to bring to a boil. Place the head of chopped bite-sized cauliflower chunks into the steamer and steam until tender, about 4 minutes. Toss the cauliflower in the bowl of dressing. Remove the steamer pan and place the bunch of chopped kale into the boiling water and continuing boiling for around 3 minutes. Drain the water and add the kale to the cauliflower, and toss to coat. Add dashes of salt and pepper and serve.

Fat Free Refried Beans

Refried beans are the perfect addition to a south-of-the-border meal. Makes 8 servings.

What You'll Need:

4 1/2 cups of water
1 1/2 cups of pinto beans (dried, sorted, rinsed)
1/4 cup of onions (chopped)
1/4 of a jalapeno pepper (seeded, finely chopped)
1 tablespoon of garlic (minced)
2 1/2 teaspoons of salt
1 teaspoon of black pepper
Pinch of cumin (ground)

How to Make It:

Add the 1 1/2 cups of pinto beans (dried, sorted, rinsed), 1/4 cup of onions (chopped), 1/4 of a jalapeno pepper (seeded, finely chopped), 1 tablespoon of garlic (minced), 2 1/2 teaspoons of salt, 1 teaspoon of black pepper, and a pinch of cumin (ground) in a slow cooker. Pour the 4 1/2 cups of water over the top. Cook on high for 8 hours, check often, and if needed add more water to make sure all the ingredients are covered. When the beans are good and tender, remove them from the liquid into a large bowl and mash them with a potato masher, adding extra liquid as needed to reach the right consistency.

Herb Roasted Potatoes

Healthier than fried potatoes, these offers a spicy taste with each bite. Makes 4 servings.

What You'll Need:

4 potatoes (large, scrubbed, peeled, cubed into bite-size)
1 tablespoon of basil (fresh chopped)
1 tablespoon of garlic (minced)
1 tablespoon of olive oil
1 tablespoon of parsley (fresh chopped)
1 tablespoon of rosemary (fresh chopped)
1/2 teaspoon of salt

How to Make It:

Prep: Preheat the oven to 475 degrees Fahrenheit. Line a baking sheet with foil.

Add the 1 tablespoon of basil (fresh chopped), 1 tablespoon of garlic (minced), 1 tablespoon of olive oil, 1 tablespoon of parsley (fresh chopped), 1 tablespoon of rosemary (fresh chopped), and 1/2 teaspoon of salt in a bowl and mix with a whisk. Add the 4 peeled and cubed potatoes and toss to coat all. Bake for 30 minutes, turning every 10 minutes. Serve immediately.

Hot 'N Spicy Black Beans

Beans make a great side dish and these give a little added flavor kick. Makes 4 servings.

What You'll Need:

1 can of black beans (15 oz., undrained)
1/2 cup of onions (chopped)
1 tablespoon of cilantro (fresh chopped)
1/2 teaspoon of garlic (minced)
1/4 teaspoon of cayenne pepper
Salt

How to Make It:

Add the 1 can of black beans (15 oz., undrained), 1/2 cup of onions (chopped), and 1/2 teaspoon of garlic (minced), to a saucepan, turn the heat to high and bring to a boil, turn to medium low and stir in the 1 tablespoon of cilantro (fresh chopped), 1/4 teaspoon of cayenne pepper, and dashes of salt. Serve immediately.

Italian Sweet Potato Fries

This is a healthier version of the French fry. Makes 4 servings.

What You'll Need:

4 sweet potatoes (peeled, cut into French fries)
2 tablespoons of olive oil
2 teaspoons of Italian seasoning
1/2 teaspoon of lemon pepper
Salt and pepper
Water

How to Make It:

Prep: Preheat the oven to 400 degrees Fahrenheit.

Place a saucepan on the stove and add the 4 French fry cut sweet potatoes, cover with water and turn to high heat. Boil for 5 minutes. Drain water and toss in the 2 tablespoons of olive oil, 2 teaspoons of Italian seasoning, 1/2 teaspoon of lemon pepper, and dashes of Salt and pepper. Spread on a baking sheet and bake for 15 minutes, flip and bake for another 15 minutes.

Lemon Garlic Broccoli

This is a roasted broccoli with lemon and garlic flavors added for a delicious side dish. Makes 6 servings.

What You'll Need:

2 broccoli heads (just the florets)
2 teaspoons of olive oil (extra virgin)
1/2 teaspoon of garlic (minced)
1/2 teaspoon of lemon juice
Salt and pepper

How to Make It:

Prep: Preheat the oven to 400 degrees Fahrenheit.

Add the florets from the 2 broccoli heads to a large bowl and toss with the 2 teaspoons of olive oil (extra virgin), 1/2 teaspoon of garlic (minced), and dashes of salt and pepper. Place in a single layer on a foil-lined baking sheet and bake until tender for about 17 minutes. Place in a serving bowl and toss with the1/2 teaspoon of lemon juice. Serve immediately.

Oven Roasted Vegetables

Here is a quick and easy way to get in a good serving of savory vegetables. Makes 6 servings.

What You'll Need:

4 potatoes (scrubbed, sliced into bite size)
1 package of frozen vegetables (10 oz. mixed)
1/2 cup of onions (chopped)
5 tablespoons of butter (divided into 10 small pats)
1 tablespoon of Italian seasoning
1 teaspoon of garlic (minced)
Salt and pepper

How to Make It:

Prep: Heat oven to 350 degrees Fahrenheit. Place 2 sheets of heavy duty foil side by side on a baking sheet, have 2 more sheets for the top. Lightly spray the foil with cooking spray on one side.

In a large bowl, combine by tossing together the 4 potatoes (scrubbed, sliced into bite size), 1 package of frozen vegetables (10 oz. mixed), 1/2 cup of onions (chopped), 1 tablespoon of Italian seasoning, 1 teaspoon of garlic (minced), and dashes of salt and pepper. Spoon equally on the center of each sheet of foil on the baking sheet. Place 5 pats of butter on top of each vegetable pile. Bring the bottom foil up to form a bowl, and place a sheet of foil on top and seal the edges, to make 2 "packets" of foil with the veggies enclosed. Bake in the oven for 15 minutes, check to make sure the potatoes are tender. Keep baking and checking every 5 minutes until the potatoes are tender enough to eat.

Potato Salad

Potato salad is a great side dish that goes with so many different main dishes. Makes 6 servings.

What You'll Need:

5 potatoes (Yukon gold)
1 cucumber (chopped, English)
2 1/2 cups of celery (chopped)
3/4 cup of onions (chopped)
3/4 cup of olives (green with pimentos, chopped)
1/2 cup of balsamic vinegar
1/4 cup of olive oil
1/4 teaspoon of garlic powder
Salt and pepper

How to Make It:

Scrub the 5 Yukon gold potatoes and place, whole, in a large saucepan. Cover the potatoes with water and turn the heat to high to bring to a boil. Turn the heat down to medium low and cook the potatoes for another 15 minutes. Drain the water and allow to cool for a few minutes. Then cut into bite sized chunks, peels and all. In a bowl, combine the cooked potatoes with the 1 cucumber (chopped, English), 2 1/2 cups of celery (chopped), 3/4 cup of onions (chopped), and the 3/4 cup of olives (green with pimentos, chopped). In a small bowl, combine the 1/2 cup of balsamic vinegar, 1/4 cup of olive oil, 1/4 teaspoon of garlic powder, and dashes of salt and pepper with a whisk. Drizzle over the potato salad and toss to coat. Refrigerate before serving. Add more salt and pepper if desired, toss again before serving.

Savory Quinoa

Quinoa is a super food packed with nutrition. It is delicious and makes a great side dish. Makes 4 servings.

What You'll Need:

2 cups of vegetable stock
1 cup of quinoa (uncooked)
1/2 cup of onions (chopped)
2 tablespoons of parsley (fresh chopped)
1 tablespoon of butter
1/2 tablespoon of thyme (fresh chopped)
2 teaspoons of garlic (minced)
Salt
Lemon juice

How to Make It:

Place the tablespoon of butter in a saucepan and turn to medium heat. Stir in the cup of uncooked quinoa, and brown for five minutes, stirring often. Add the 2 cups of vegetable stock and turn heat to high to bring to a boil. Reduce heat to low and simmer for 15 minutes with a lid to cover. Check to see if the quinoa is tender, if not, keep cooking until it becomes tender. Add the cooked quinoa in a bowl and toss in the 1/2 cup of onions (chopped), 2 tablespoons of parsley (fresh chopped), 1 tablespoon of butter, 1/2 tablespoon of thyme (fresh chopped), 2 teaspoons of garlic (minced), and dashes of salt and lemon juice. Serve immediately.

Spicy Pinto Beans

Take your average pot of pinto beans and turn up the heat, way up! Makes 8 servings.

What You'll Need:

1 lb. of pinto beans (dried)
1 jalapeno (fine chopped)
3 2/3 cup of chicken stock
3/4 cup of onions (chopped)
1/2 cup of green salsa
1 teaspoon of cumin (ground)
1 teaspoon of garlic (minced)
Salt and pepper
Water

How to Make It:

Prep: Sort, rinse, and soak the beans overnight.

Combine the 1 lb. of pinto beans (dried), 1 jalapeno (fine chopped), 3 2/3 cup of chicken stock, 3/4 cup of onions (chopped), 1/2 cup of green salsa, 1 teaspoon of cumin (ground), 1 teaspoon of garlic (minced), and dashes of salt and pepper in a large pan on the stove. Turn to high heat and bring to a boil. Turn to medium low and cook until the beans are tender, about 2 hours. Add more water if needed.

Spicy Roasted Baked Potatoes

This is a delicious combination of spicy and sweet.
Makes 4 servings.

What You'll Need:

3 sweet potatoes (large, washed, peeled, and cut into
chunks)
2 tablespoons of olive oil
Dried oregano
Salt and Pepper

How to Make It:

Prep: Preheat the oven to 350 degrees Fahrenheit. Line
a baking sheet with foil and spray it with cooking spray.

Place the sweet potatoes in a large bowl, toss in 2
tablespoons of olive oil. Sprinkle the dried oregano, salt,
and pepper and toss again so that all pieces are coated
with oil and seasonings. Spread the chunks out onto a
baking sheet and bake for at least an hour, until they are
tender. Serve immediately.

Tangy Vegetable Salad

This is a delicious side dish or a night light lunch. Makes 8 servings.

What You'll Need:

3 cans of corn (11 oz., whole kernel)
4 scallions (chopped)
2 tomatoes (diced)
1 bunch of cilantro (fresh chopped)
3/4 cup of onions (thin sliced)
1/3 cup of rice vinegar
Salt

How to Make It:

Combine the 3 cans of corn (11 oz., whole kernel), 4 scallions (chopped), 2 tomatoes (diced), 1 bunch of cilantro (fresh chopped), and 3/4 cup of onions (thin sliced), tossing. Drizzle and toss the 1/3 cup of rice vinegar and a couple dashes of salt. Refrigerate for about 30 to 45 minutes. Toss again prior to serving.

Eating Clean Main Dish Recipes

Baked Italian Crusted Cod

Cod is nutritious and a good way to get in the weekly fish you should be eating. The cod has an Italian crust that tastes fried even though it was baked. Makes 4 servings.

What You'll Need:

4 cod fillets
1/4 cup of bread crumbs (from whole grain bread)
1 egg white
2 tablespoons of Parmesan cheese (grated)
1 tablespoon of cornmeal
1 teaspoon of olive oil
1/2 teaspoon of Italian seasoning
1/2 teaspoon of garlic (minced)
1/8 teaspoon of black pepper (ground)

How to Make It:

Prep: Preheat the oven to 450 degrees Fahrenheit.

Combine the 1/4 cup of bread crumbs (from whole grain

bread), 2 tablespoons of Parmesan cheese (grated), 1 tablespoon of cornmeal, 1 teaspoon of olive oil, 1/2 teaspoon of Italian seasoning, 1/2 teaspoon of garlic (minced), and 1/8 teaspoon of black pepper (ground) in a bowl. Spray a boiler pan with cooking spray. Place the cod on the boiler pan. Beat the egg white slightly, and then brush onto the tops of the cod fillets. Evenly divide the breadcrumb mixture onto the tops of the cod. Bake until the fish is done, when it flakes apart, about 11 minutes.

Balsamic Chicken and Rice.

This savory chicken dish is an excellent companion with a side dish of rice. Makes 6 servings.

What You'll Need:

6 chicken breast halves (boneless, skinless)
1 can of tomatoes (14.5 oz., diced)
1/2 cup of onion (thin sliced)
1/2 cup of balsamic vinegar
2 tablespoons of olive oil
1 teaspoon of garlic salt
1 teaspoon of basil (dried)
1 teaspoon of oregano (dried)
1 teaspoon of rosemary (dried)
1/2 teaspoon of thyme (dried)
Black pepper
Rice (cooked, enough for 6 servings)

How to Make It:

Sprinkle the teaspoon of garlic salt and a couple of dashes of black pepper on the 6 boneless, skinless chicken breast halves. Add the 2 tablespoons of olive oil to a skillet and heat to medium high and cooked the chicken breasts and sauté the 1/2 cup of thin sliced onion. Add the can of 14.5 oz. can of diced tomatoes and the 1/2 cup of balsamic vinegar over the chicken. Stir in the 1 teaspoon of basil (dried), 1 teaspoon of oregano (dried), 1 teaspoon of rosemary (dried), and 1/2 teaspoon of thyme (dried). Cooking for about 15 minutes, until the chicken turns solid white. Serve a breast half over a spoon of cooked rice.

Basic Spaghetti Sauce

This is a savory, delicious sauce that tastes great over chicken, homemade pasta, eggplants, vegetables, or wherever spaghetti sauce is used. Makes 8 servings.

What You'll Need:

2 cans of tomato sauce (15 oz. each)
1 can of tomatoes (14.5 oz., stewed)
1 can of tomato paste (6 oz.)
4 mushrooms (fresh, sliced)
1 bell pepper (green ,chopped)
1/2 cup of onion (chopped)
1 tablespoon of olive oil
1 1/2 teaspoons of garlic (minced)
1/4 teaspoon of basil (dried)
1/4 teaspoon of oregano (dried)
Black pepper

How to Make It:

Add the tablespoon of olive oil to a skillet and turn to medium heat. Sauté the 1 bell pepper (green ,chopped), 1/2 cup of onion (chopped), and the 1 1/2 teaspoons of garlic (minced). Stir in the 1/4 teaspoon of basil (dried), 1/4 teaspoon of oregano (dried), and dashes of black pepper. Add the 14.5 oz. can of stewed tomatoes and cook until the sauce thickens. Add the 2 15 oz. cans of tomato sauce and the 6 oz. can of tomato paste. Turn heat to low, stir and simmer for 15 minutes.

Beefy Chili

This is a tried and true traditional chili recipe. Makes 8 servings.

What You'll Need:

1 pound of ground beef (lean)
2 cans of tomato puree (10.75 oz.)
2 cans of kidney beans (15 oz. each, 1 undrained and 1 drained)
1 can of cannellini beans (15 oz., undrained)
3/4 cup of onions (diced)
3/4 cup of celery (dice)
3/4 cup of bell pepper (green, diced)
1/2 tablespoon of chili powder
1 teaspoon of garlic (minced)
3/4 teaspoon of basil (dried)
3/4 teaspoon of oregano (dried)
1/2 teaspoon of parsley (dried)
Couple shakes of hot pepper sauce
Salt and pepper

How to Make It:

Cook the pound of lean ground beef over medium high heat in a skillet. Drain off grease. Add the cooked beef to a slow cooker followed by 2 cans of tomato puree (10.75 oz.), 2 cans of kidney beans (15 oz. each, 1 undrained and 1 drained), 1 can of cannellini beans (15 oz., undrained), 3/4 cup of onions (diced), 3/4 cup of celery (dice), 3/4 cup of bell pepper (green, diced), 1/2 tablespoon of chili powder, 1 teaspoon of garlic (minced), 3/4 teaspoon of basil (dried), 3/4 teaspoon of oregano (dried), 1/2 teaspoon of parsley (dried), a couple shakes of hot pepper sauce, and dashes of salt and pepper. Stir, cover, and cook on low for eight hours or on high for four hours.

Chicken Chili

This is a bowl of delicious spicy chicken chili, the perfect comfort food. Makes 4 servings.

What You'll Need:

4 chicken breasts (halves, boneless, skinless, cubed)
1 can of cannellini beans (15 oz., drained, rinsed)
1 can of green chilies (4 oz., diced)
2 green onions (chopped)
1 1/4 cups of chicken stock
1/2 cup of Monterey Jack cheese (shredded)
1/2 cup of onion (chopped)
1 tablespoon of olive oil
1 teaspoon of garlic powder
1 teaspoon of cumin (ground)
1/2 teaspoon of cilantro (dried)
1/2 teaspoon of oregano (dried)
1/8 teaspoon of cayenne pepper

How to Make It:

Add the tablespoon of olive oil to a large size saucepan and turn to medium high heat. Add the 4 chicken breasts (halves, boneless, skinless, cubed) and the 1/2 cup of chopped onions and cook for 5 minutes, while stirring. Pour in the 1 1/4 cups of chicken stock and add the 1 can of green chilies (4 oz., diced), 1 teaspoon of garlic powder, 1 teaspoon of cumin (ground), 1/2 teaspoon of cilantro (dried), 1/2 teaspoon of oregano (dried), and the 1/8 teaspoon of cayenne pepper. Turn the heat to low and cook for 15 minutes. Add the 1 can of cannellini beans (15 oz., drained, rinsed) and cook until the chicken is well done and white about another five minutes. Ladle into bowls and divide the 2 chopped green onions and the 1/2 cup of shredded Monterey Jack cheese on top.

Cod and Salsa

This is a delicious spicy cod, if you want it hot use a hotter salsa. Makes 4 servings.

What You'll Need:

1.5 pounds of cod fillets (rinse and pat dry)
2 cups of salsa
2 tablespoons of parsley (fresh chopped)
Lemon juice
Salt and pepper
Rice (cooked, 4 servings)

How to Make It:

Prep: Preheat the oven to 350 degrees Fahrenheit. Line a baking dish with foil and lightly spray with cooking spray.

Sprinkle the 2 tablespoons of fresh chopped parsley, lemon juice, and dashes of salt and pepper over the cod. Bake until flaky for about half an hour. Serve each serving over a serving of cooked rice.

Fruit Salsa Salmon

This is a deliciously sweet and spicy salmon dish, perfect over a bed of rice. Makes 4 servings.

What You'll Need:

1 pound of salmon steaks
Rice (cooked, enough for 4 servings)
2 jalapeno peppers (diced)
1 tomato (diced)
1 lemon (sliced)
1/2 cup of pineapple juice
1/3 cup of water
1/4 cup of bell pepper (red, diced)
1/4 cup of bell pepper (yellow, diced)
1/4 cup of pineapple (fresh diced)
1/4 cup of onion (minced)
2 tablespoons of lemon juice
1 tablespoon of rosemary (fresh chopped)
1 1/2 teaspoons of garlic (minced)
Salt and pepper

How to Make It:

Prep: Preheat the oven to 350 degrees Fahrenheit.

Place the salmon steaks in a shallow baking pan, sprinkle the 2 tablespoons of lemon juice over the top. Sprinkle with the 1 tablespoon of rosemary (fresh chopped) and dashes of salt and pepper. Cover with slices of the lemon. Add the 1/3 cup of water to the pan. Bake for 40 minutes, after the water evaporates and the fish is flakey it is done. In a bowl, make the fruit salsa by combining the 2 jalapeno peppers (diced), 1 tomato (diced), 1/2 cup of pineapple juice,
1/3 cup of water, 1/4 cup of bell pepper (red, diced), 1/4 cup of bell pepper (yellow, diced), 1/4 cup of pineapple (fresh diced), 1/4 cup of onion (minced), 1 tablespoon of rosemary (fresh chopped), and 1 1/2 teaspoons of garlic (minced). Divide the salmon steaks into 4 servings. Add a serving of rice on the plate, top with a salmon steak, and then 1/4 of the fruit salsa. Serve immediately.

Glazed Salmon

Here is a delicious spicy hot and sweet glazed salmon.
Makes 4 servings.

What You'll Need:

1 salmon filet (.75 pound, skinless)
1 1/2 cups of apricot nectar
1/3 cup of apricots (chopped, dried)
2 tablespoons of honey
2 tablespoons of soy sauce
1 tablespoon of ginger (fresh grated)
1 teaspoon of garlic (minced)
1/4 teaspoon of cinnamon (ground)
1/8 teaspoon of cayenne pepper

How to Make It:

Prep: Preheat the boiler on high. Spray the boiler pan
with cooking spray.

Combine the 1 1/2 cups of apricot nectar, 1/3 cup of
apricots (chopped, dried), 2 tablespoons of honey, 2
tablespoons of soy sauce, 1 tablespoon of ginger (fresh
grated), 1 teaspoon of garlic (minced), 1/4 teaspoon of
cinnamon (ground), and the 1/8 teaspoon of cayenne

pepper in a saucepan over medium heat, stirring often until it comes to a boil. Turn to medium low and cook for 20 minutes. Stir often to prevent sticking and burning. Pull out 1/4 cup of liquid and set aside. Put the salmon filet on the prepared boiler pan. Brush with the glaze in the saucepan. Place under the boiler for 8 minutes. Then baste ever minute for 4 more minutes. Remove from oven, serve with the reserved glaze.

Grilled Turkey Breast

This is a delicious dish of seasoned savory turkey breast. Makes about 10 servings.

What You'll Need:

2 turkey breast (boneless, halves)
1/4 cup of canola oil
1/4 cup of soy sauce
6 cloves (whole)
2 tablespoons of lemon juice
1 tablespoon of honey
1 tablespoon of basil (fresh chopped)
1 teaspoon of garlic (minced)
1/2 teaspoon of black pepper (ground)

How to Make It:

First, combine the 1 tablespoon of basil (fresh chopped), 1 teaspoon of garlic (minced), and the 1/2 teaspoon of black pepper (ground). This is the rub, wash and pat dry the boneless turkey breast halves, then rub into each one. In a separate bowl, combine the 1/4 cup of canola oil, 1/4 cup of soy sauce, 2 tablespoons of lemon juice, and the 1 tablespoon of honey. Coat the turkey breast halves in the marinade. Arrange them in a baking dish and place the 6 cloves all around the breasts. Seal with foil and refrigerate for four hours. Turn the grill to high. Spray the grate with cooking spray. Grill the turkey breasts on the hot grill, lid closed, for 30 minutes, flipping half way through. Check to make sure the internal temperature reaches 170 degrees Fahrenheit.

Honey Mustard Chicken

This is recipe is a favorite for young and old alike. Makes 6 servings.

What You'll Need:

6 chicken breast halves (boneless, skinless)
1/2 cup of honey
1/2 cup of yellow prepared mustard
1 teaspoon of basil (dried)
1 teaspoon of paprika
1/2 teaspoon of parsley (dried)
Salt and pepper

How to Make It:

Prep: Preheat the oven to 350 degrees Fahrenheit. Line a 9x13 inch baking dish with foil and lightly spray with cooking spray.

Rinse and dry the 6 boneless, skinless chicken breast halves and sprinkle with dash of salt and pepper. Lay the chicken in the prepared baking dish. Make the sauce by combining the 1/2 cup of honey, 1/2 cup of yellow prepared mustard, 1 teaspoon of basil (dried), 1 teaspoon of paprika, and 1/2 teaspoon of parsley (dried) in a bowl with a whisk. Brush on all sides of the seasoned chicken breasts. Bake in the hot oven for 15 minutes. Turn the oven off and let sit in the cooling oven for 10 minutes before serving.

Italian Parmesan Eggplant

This delicious dish uses the Basic Spaghetti Sauce recipe as well, making a delightful Italian dish. Makes 8 servings.

What You'll Need:

12 slices of whole grain bread
3 eggplants (peeled, sliced thin)
2 eggs
6 cups of spaghetti sauce (use the Basic Spaghetti Sauce recipe)
4 cups of mozzarella cheese (shredded, divided)
1/2 cup of Parmesan cheese (grated, divided)
1/2 teaspoon of basil (dried)
Italian seasoning
Olive oil (to drizzle)

How to Make It:

First, make the breadcrumbs. Take the 12 slices of whole grain bread and drizzle olive oil over them, then give about 2 shakes of the Italian seasoning. Place them on a baking sheet and place under a hot boiler until they are toasted to a light golden brown, a couple of minutes. Flip over and repeat the above. Remove from oven and set aside to cool. When cooled, cut into fine "bread crumbs." You can put into a food processor for a few seconds to make the fine breadcrumbs.

Preheat the oven to 350 degrees Fahrenheit. In a bowl beat the 2 eggs with a whisk. Dip each slice of eggplant in the eggs, then in the fine breadcrumbs. Pour the 6 cups of spaghetti sauce into a 9x13 inch baking pan. Place half of the crusted eggplant slices in the bottom; sprinkle 2 cups of shredded mozzarella cheese and 1/4 cup of grated Parmesan Cheese. Repeat the layers and then sprinkle the 1/2 teaspoon of dried basil over the top. Bake until a nice crusty golden brown, about 35 minutes.

Mexican Chicken

This delicious chicken meal satisfies those south of the border cravings. Makes 4 servings.

What You'll Need:

4 servings of cooked rice
4 chicken breast halves (boneless, skinless)
1 can of black beans (15 oz., drained, rinsed)
1 can of tomatoes with green chili peppers (diced, 10 oz.)
1 can of corn (whole kernels, 8.75 oz., drained)
1 tablespoon of canola oil
Pinch of cumin (ground)

How to Make It:

Add the tablespoon of canola oil to a large skillet and turn to medium high. Cook the 4 boneless, skinless chicken breast halves until lightly browned on all sides. Stir in the 1 can of black beans (15 oz., drained, rinsed), 1 can of tomatoes with green chili peppers (diced, 10 oz.), and the 1 can of corn (whole kernels, 8.75 oz., drained). Turn the heat to medium low and simmer for half an hour. Add the pinch of ground cumin prior to serving over a bed of rice.

Orange Lime Shrimp

This is a tangy shrimp recipe that is simple to make and delicious to eat. Serve with vegetables and rice.

What You'll Need:

1 1/2 pounds of shrimp (peeled, deveined, large)
2/3 cup of orange juice
1/3 cup of lime juice
2 tablespoons of orange zest
2 tablespoons of olive oil
1 tablespoon of lime zest
1 1/2 teaspoon of garlic (minced)
1/2 teaspoon of salt

How to Make It:

Add the 2/3 cup of orange juice, 1/3 cup of lime juice, 2 tablespoons of orange zest, 2 tablespoons of olive oil, 1 tablespoon of lime zest, 1 1/2 teaspoon of garlic (minced), and 1/2 teaspoon of salt to a blender or food processor and blend until smooth. Pour into a bowl and toss in the 1 1/2 pounds of peeled deveined shrimp and let sit for 20 minutes, on the countertop. Place a non-stick skillet on the stove and turn to medium high. Cook each shrimp for several minutes until it turns opaque.

Baste with the marinade while they cook. Serve immediately.

Orange Roughy

This is a different twist for orange roughy with a touch of lemon and orange. Makes 4 servings.

What You'll Need:

4 orange roughy fillets
2 tablespoons of orange juice
2 tablespoons of lemon juice
1 tablespoon of olive oil
1/2 teaspoon of lemon pepper

How to Make It:

Place the tablespoon of olive oil in a skillet and heat to medium high. Add the 4 orange roughy fillets and cook for a couple of minutes, then drizzle with the 2 tablespoons of orange juice and the 2 tablespoons of lemon juice. Sprinkle with the 1/2 teaspoon of lemon pepper. Cook until the fish is flaky.

Spicy Black Beans and Quinoa

This is a delicious dish filled with super foods, packed with nutrition and flavor.

What You'll Need:

2 cans of black beans (15 oz., drained, rinsed)
1 1/2 cups of vegetable stock
1 cup of corn (frozen)
3/4 cup of quinoa (uncooked)
1/2 cup of cilantro (fresh chopped)
1/2 cup of onion (chopped)
1 1/2 teaspoons of garlic (minced)
1 teaspoon of cumin (ground)
1 teaspoon of canola oil
1/4 teaspoon of cayenne pepper
Salt and pepper

How to Make It:

Pour the teaspoon of canola oil in mid-sized saucepan and heat to medium. Add the 1/2 cup of chopped onions and the 1 1/2 teaspoons of minced garlic and sauté. Stir in the 3/4 cup of uncooked quinoa and the 1 1/2 cups of vegetable stock. Sprinkle in the 1 teaspoon of cumin (ground), 1 teaspoon of canola oil, 1/4 teaspoon of cayenne pepper, and dashes of salt and pepper. Turn the heat to high and bring to a boil. Cover and reduce to low and simmer for about 20 minutes. Add the cup of frozen corn, stir, and cook for another 5 minutes. Add the 2 15 oz. cans of drained, rinsed black beans and the 1/2 cup of fresh chopped cilantro. Cook until heated through and serve.

Sweet and Tangy Tilapia

Fish lovers will enjoy this sweet and tangy tilapia. Makes 4 servings.

What You'll Need:

1 pound of tilapia (fillets)
1 butternut squash (sliced)
1 bunch of asparagus (fresh, trimmed)
1/2 cup of mozzarella cheese (shredded)
1/4 cup of honey
3 tablespoons of lime juice
1 teaspoon of garlic (minced)
Salt and pepper
Poultry seasoning

How to Make It:

Combine the 1/4 cup of honey, 3 tablespoons of lime juice, and 1 teaspoon of garlic (minced) in a bowl. Sprinkle salt and pepper on the tilapia and add to the marinade, turning the fish to coat. Refrigerate for an hour.

Preheat the oven to 350 degrees Fahrenheit. Spray a baking dish (large enough to lay the tilapia in) with cooking spray. Add the sliced butternut squash and the fresh trimmed asparagus in the bottom of the baking dish. Place the marinated fish on top. Sprinkle with dashes of poultry seasoning. Bake in the hot oven until the fish is flaky and the vegetables are tender, about 20 minutes. Add the 1/2 cup of shredded mozzarella cheese on top and bake another 5 minutes, until the cheese melts. Serve immediately.

Tuna Salad

This is a refreshingly light main dish, makes a perfect lunch too. Makes 4 servings.

What You'll Need:

2 cans of tuna (6oz, packed in water, drained)
2 scallions (chopped)
1 apple (cored, cut into bite sizes)
8 cups of spinach (fresh chopped)
2/3 cup of cranberries (dried)
1/4 cup of mayonnaise
Salt and pepper

How to Make It:

Combine the 2 cans of tuna (6oz, packed in water, drained), 2 scallions (chopped), 1 apple (cored, cut into bite sizes), 2/3 cup of cranberries (dried), 1/4 cup of mayonnaise, and dashes of salt and pepper in a bowl. Divide the 8 cups of spinach (fresh chopped) in 4 plates. Divide the tuna salad over the fresh chopped spinach and serve.

1Turkey Chili

This is another version of a delicious comfort food made with chili. Makes 6 servings.

What You'll Need:

1.5 lbs. of ground turkey
1 bell pepper (green, chopped)
1 can of tomatoes (28 oz., diced)
1 can of black beans (19 oz., drained)
1 can of corn (15.25 oz., whole kernel, undrained)
Dashes of chili powder
Dashes of cinnamon (ground)
Dashes of cumin (ground)
Dashes of red pepper flakes

How to Make It:

Cook the 1.5 lbs. of ground turkey in a skillet on medium heat. Transfer the browned ground turkey to a large saucepan and add the 1 bell pepper (green, chopped), 1 can of tomatoes (28 oz., diced), 1 can of black beans (19 oz., drained), 1 can of corn (15.25 oz., whole kernel, undrained), dashes of chili powder , dashes of cinnamon (ground), dashes of cumin (ground), and dashes of red pepper flakes. Stir and turn the heat to high to bring to a boil. Reduce heat to simmer for half an hour.

Turkey Meatloaf

Turkey is a good lean meat and if you love meatloaf, you will love this recipe. Makes 5 servings.

What You'll Need:

1/2 pound of ground turkey
1 egg
1/2 cup of salsa (divided)
1/4 cup of onions (chopped)
1/4 cup of bread crumbs (from whole grain bread)
1/8 cup of bell pepper (chopped red)
1/8 cup of bell pepper (chopped yellow)

How to Make It:

Prep: Preheat the oven to 350 degrees Fahrenheit. Line a loaf pan with foil and lightly spray with cooking spray.

Add the 1/2 pound of ground turkey, 1 egg, 1/4 cup of salsa, 1/4 cup of onions (chopped), 1/4 cup of bread crumbs (from whole grain bread), 1/8 cup of bell pepper (chopped red), and 1/8 cup of bell pepper (chopped yellow) and mix with bare hands. Mold into a loaf and place in the loaf pan. Pour the remaining 1/4 cup of salsa over the top and bake until well done, when a meat thermometer reaches 165 degrees Fahrenheit, about 25 minutes.

Section 2: Belly Fat Diet

Even if you have lost weight and you have toned up your body, you may still be dealing with stubborn belly fat. Belly fat is difficult to lose. You may be working out and trying to eat right, but it may seem that your belly just refuses to get flatter. If this is a problem you are dealing with, the belly fat diet may be the right diet for your needs. This diet is specifically designed to help you lose belly fat now. The foods included in the diet help target belly fat, helping you finally get rid of that belly.

This book is packed with all the information you need to successfully follow the belly fat diet and lose belly fat now. You will find helpful information on the diet, the benefits of following this diet and more. As you get started on the diet, you can enjoy using some of the helpful tips provided to ensure you are successful when you begin using this diet. The best part of this book is the many powerful recipes that will help support your belly melt diet. You will not have to start searching for recipes that go with your new diet.

Recipes are included for every meal. Great breakfast recipes will help you start out your day the right way. Tasty lunch recipes will keep you fueled up during the day and help you avoid cravings. The dinner recipes included will help you enjoy tasty meals that even your family will enjoy and many of them are ready in only a short amount of time, allowing you to add healthy eating to your busy life. You may be surprised to find dessert and snack recipes as well. Enjoy a delicious dessert or snack without sabotaging your belly fat diet.

You can finally get rid of that belly you have had for so long. Use these tips and the delicious recipes and included and you will quickly be on your way to a flatter belly.

Chapter 1: What is the Belly Fat Diet?

What is the belly fat diet? Maybe you have heard about this diet but you are not quite sure what it is and how it works. Basically, the belly fat diet is a special diet that is designed to help you take off inches of belly fat. You will lose weight while you are on this diet. However, the important part to note is that you will be taking off belly fat, not just losing a few pounds. While every individual is difference, most people end up losing 12-15 pounds within a month when they follow this diet. Several inches of belly fat are usually lost as well. The great thing about the diet is that you will not have to do hundreds of crunches to enjoy a flatter belly.

The Secret Behind the Diet

There is one big secret behind the diet – MUFAs. What are MUFAs? They are monounsaturated fatty acids. These fatty acids work to eliminate belly fat and they also make you feel full. Not only will you melt away belly fat when adding MUFAs to your diet, but these fatty acids will keep you feeling satisfied, which can help keep you from overeating as well. MUFAs are plant based fats and they can be found in foods like olive oil, chocolate, seeds, avocados and nuts. To get the best results while on this diet, you should strive to get a serving of MUFAs with every meal that you eat.

Even though MUFAs are fatty acids, these are healthy fats. They will not clog up your arteries. Instead, they actually help to improve your health. Along with the emphasis on MUFAs, which is the big secret behind this diet, the diet also emphasizes eating key foods like whole grains, fish, veggies, fruits, legumes and olive oil. In fact, this diet includes foods that are often found within the Mediterranean approach to eating.

How the Diet Works

Now that you know the secret behind the diet, you may be wondering how the diet works. The diet focuses on eating about 1600 calories a day and also involves eating a serving of MUFAs with each meal that you eat. Of course, keep in mind that you can tailor the number of calories you take in to your gender, activity level and your age. The diet includes avoiding processed, high fat foods. While protein is an important part of each meal, the focus is on vegetables and fruits with each meal.

The great thing about this diet is that most people find it very easy to follow. While you will have to restrict your diet to some extent, you still are able to enjoy wonderful meals that include delicious dishes. Many of the recipes included with this diet are easy to prepare, which makes this diet easy to follow, even for individuals that are very busy. You will not have to worry about skimping on taste either. Enjoy chocolate dishes, veggie pizzas and other great recipes that are sure to keep your taste buds happy.

Chapter 2: Benefits of the Belly Fat Diet

Belly fat, while it can be unsightly, can actually have serious long term health consequences. While going on the belly fat diet can help you lose your belly and feel better about the way you look, the main benefits of losing belly fat are health benefits. Unfortunately, while belly fat can be so dangerous, it is also extremely difficult to lose. Going on the belly fat diet can help blast away that belly fat. While you may already be excited about trying this diet, here are a few of the top benefits you can enjoy with this diet, which may excite you even more.

Benefit #1 – Reduce the Risk of Diabetes and Heart Disease

One of the best benefits of going on the belly fat diet is that it can help to reduce your risk of diabetes and heart disease. Excess belly fat can drastically increase your risk of developing diseases like diabetes and heart disease. In fact, excess belly fat can be almost as dangerous as smoking when it comes to increasing your risk of diseases like heart disease. The great news is that you can eliminate belly fat as a major risk factor for diabetes and heart disease. By following the belly fat diet, you can reduce your belly fat and begin reducing your risk of dealing with diabetes or heart disease in the future. In fact, your overall health will be improved as you melt that belly fat away.

Benefit #2 – Keep Testosterone Levels Normal

Studies show that having too much belly fat may lead to a reduction in testosterone within the body. This is especially troublesome for men, although women have testosterone as well. Low testosterone in men often causes impotence and lack of libido. The good news is that losing that belly fat can help keep testosterone at normal levels. Eliminating belly fat naturally begins to bring up testosterone levels. Adding exercise to the belly fat diet will boost levels of testosterone even more.

Benefit #3 – Enjoy Better Sleep at Night

Newer research that was done by Johns Hopkins shows that those who have more belly fat may not sleep as well as those with little belly fat. Losing belly fat may actually improve sleep quality. The study showed that those who reduced abdominal fat actually improved their sleep quality assessment test scores. This is important, since lack of sleep can cause a range of different health problems, including heart disease, depression and more. Simply losing some belly fat may be enough to help you sleep better, avoiding chronic lack of sleep.

Benefit #4 – Feel Better About Yourself

Last, the belly fat diet can help you blast away that troublesome belly fat, which has the benefit of helping you feel better about yourself. You may have a negative self-image of yourself while you still have belly fat. Losing the belly fat can help you improve your self-image, becoming happier with the way you look and feel. You may also enjoy feeling satisfied and triumphant when you succeed at improving your body and your health with the belly fat diet.

Chapter 3: Essential Tips for Success on the Belly Melt Diet

As you begin your belly fat diet, you want to ensure that you are successful. It can be easy to let a busy life get you off track when you are on a diet or to fall back into old habits that sabotage your efforts. To help you make the most of this diet, we have put together some great diet tips that will boost your belly melting efforts. You will also find a closer look at some of the top belly fat burning foods that you can work to add to this diet on a regular basis. With this information to guide you, you will have no problem making this diet successful.

Helpful Diet Tips to Follow

While the belly fat diet focuses on reducing calories, adding MUFAs and eating wholesome foods, there are some other tips you can follow to make the most of this diet. To help you get better results as you work to lose that belly fat, here are some helpful diet tips you definitely want to follow as you go on the belly fat diet.

- **Tip #1 – Avoid Drinking Your Calories** – On the belly fat diet, you should be taking in about 1600 calories each day. One of your best tips for success is to avoid drinking your calories. You may be surprised to find that many tasty drinks like shakes, juices and some coffee beverages can have hundreds of calories in a single drink. This quickly takes a big bite out of the calories you are supposed to have each day. Another big problem is that most of the calories in these drinks come from sugar, which can actually make your body store more belly fat instead of losing it. Instead of drinking your calories, focus on drinking plenty of water. You can also drink black coffee and certain teas without adding calories to your diet. Making this one simple change to your diet as you take on the belly fat diet can make a huge difference and help you lose that belly fat faster.

- **Tip #2 – Stay Away From Anything Processed and Refined** – Another helpful diet tip to follow while you are on the belly melt diet is to stay away from anything that is processed and refined. Processed foods usually have their nutrients stripped away when they are refined. They may also include many additives and sugar. That added sugar can make you feel hungrier, lead to more fat storage and can increase the production of insulin within your body. Processed, refined foods will sabotage your belly fat diet. Stay away from them and you are sure to enjoy better results.

- **Tip #3 – Don't Be Afraid to Cheat Once a Week –** It can be difficult to stick to a new diet all the time, especially if you are craving a specific food that you cannot have on your new diet. To make sure you stick with this belly fat diet, do not be afraid to cheat once a week. On one day, allow yourself to have one dessert that you have been craving or let yourself eat one cheeseburger or a slice of pizza. Knowing that you can cheat once a week can help you stick to your diet during the rest of the week. Feeling deprived can make you fail at your diet. Instead of feeling deprived, remind yourself that once each week you can enjoy cheating for a meal. It will go a long way towards helping you stick with the belly fat diet as you blast that fat away for good.

Top Belly Fat Burning Foods

While MUFAs are one of the big secrets to this belly fat diet, there are many other great belly fat burning foods that you can add to your diet to help you melt that belly fat. Here is a look at some of the top belly fat burning foods you should be eating and information on why they help you eliminate belly fat.

- **Fruits Rich in Fiber** – It is important to have plenty of fruits in your diet, especially those that are rich in fiber. They help make sure you get all the vitamins and minerals that your body needs. Berries are particularly important, since they are high in antioxidants and will help blast away belly fat. Some of the other great fruits that you should eat while on this diet include papayas, oranges, watermelon, peaches, cantaloupes, apples and apricots. Just make sure you eat fruits raw instead of drinking fruit juices.

- **Fiber Rich Veggies** – Veggies are an important part of your belly fat diet and they help make sure your body is burning off fat effectively. Some of the best vegies include leafy greens like cabbage, kale, lettuces and spinach. Other great veggies include cucumbers, broccoli, tomatoes and zucchini. Veggies can be eaten in salads, added to soups, stir fried, steamed or added to other dishes. The great thing about fiber rich veggies is that they fill you up and help to fight off cravings, which helps make it easier to lose belly fat.

- **Eggs** – Eggs are a powerful belly fat burning food to eat while following the belly fat diet. They have important vitamins that help your body burn fat. Eggs also have a lot of protein, which keeps you feeling full as well. Poach eggs, scramble them or even eat them hard boiled. They make a great breakfast that will fuel you for your day and help boost your belly melting efforts.

- **Green Tea** – Adding green tea to your belly fat diet is a great idea for several reasons. First, it works by flushing toxins out of your body naturally, eliminating water retention and bloating. It also has compounds that are known to help with weight loss, giving your metabolism a boost. Add a bit of lemon juice and honey to the tea for a very low calorie drink that will help burn fat.

- **Beans** – Different types of beans are a great addition to your belly fat diet as well. Beans are very high in protein, which can help to blast away stomach fat. Some great beans to try include Edamame, garbanzo beans, chick peas, kidney beans and black beans. Of course, when you add beans to your diet, avoid consuming them in large amounts. Too many beans can lead to bloating and gas, which will make your belly feel bigger.

These are just a few of the excellent foods that should be included in your belly fat diet. Along with the addition of MUFAs, they can help to blast away belly fat, helping you to enjoy success as you take on this new diet plan.

Chapter 4: Belly Melting Breakfast Recipes

Breakfast is the most important meal of your day, especially when you are trying to lose belly fat. On the belly fat diet, you need to make sure you get a good breakfast in your stomach to keep you feeling full until lunch. These recipes are packed with protein, fiber and healthy fats, helping you feel satisfied while ensuring you enjoy what you're eating.

Banana Walnut Breakfast Muffin Recipe

These delicious muffins make any breakfast special, including all the flavors you'd expect to find in a banana split. The great thing about these muffins is that they are perfect for your belly fat diet too. Breakfast will almost feel like dessert when you make these muffins for breakfast. In fact, you may want to make a few extras and freeze them to enjoy at a later date.

What You'll Need:

¾ cup of mini chocolate chips, semisweet

1 ½ cups of walnuts, chopped

¼ cup of canola oil

1 banana, very ripe and mashed

½ cup of dark brown sugar, packed

1 ½ cups of all-purpose flour

1 large egg

¼ cup of Greek yogurt, plain

½ teaspoon of ground cinnamon

¼ cup of skim milk

1 teaspoon of vanilla

1 tablespoon of baking powder

½ teaspoon of salt

How to Make It:

Start by preheating the oven to 375F. Add muffin papers to a muffin pan or use cooking spray to prepare a 12 cup muffin pan.

Add a half cup of walnuts to a food processor, processing until you have a very find powder. Next, place the freshly ground walnuts, baking powder, salt, flour, cinnamon, and chocolate chips in a large mixing bowl. Mix and combine thoroughly.

In a medium sized mixing bowl, combine the milk, vanilla, oil, egg, brown sugar, banana and yogurt. Stir until the mixture becomes smooth. Combine the flour and banana mixtures together, combining well. Last, stir the last cup of chopped walnuts into the batter. The batter should be quite thick.

Fill each muffin cup with the batter until about ¾ of the way full. Place muffins in the oven, allowing to bake for about 15 minutes. Check muffins for doneness. If the tops lightly spring back when you touch them, they are done. Remove muffins from the oven. Allow to sit for a few minutes. Then, remove each muffin from the muffin tin, placing them on a rack to cool. Makes 12 muffins.

Tomato Pesto Eggs Florentine Breakfast Recipe

A recipe from Prevention.com inspires this tasty recipe. It is easy to make, even for those who have never poached eggs in the past. While this recipe is wonderful for any breakfast, it makes a wonderful dish to serve guests for a nice brunch. It offers a nice mixture of protein, carbs and veggies, getting you ready for your shape. The bit of vinegar added to the recipe helps the egg whites to keep their shape while cooking.

What You'll Need:

1/3 cup of Greek yogurt, fat free
4 large eggs
1 teaspoon of olive oil
1 teaspoon of vinegar
1 9-oz package of baby spinach, prewashed
2 English muffins, whole grain, split and then toasted
¼ cup of sun-dried tomato pesto
Ground black pepper, freshly ground
Pinch of salt

How to Make It:

In a large skillet, heat up the olive oil on medium heat. One oil is hot, add spinach to the pan, cooking it just until it wilts. In a small bowl, combine the sun-dried tomato pesto and the yogurt. Then, stir a ¼ cup of the mixture into the spinach, immediate removing the spinach from the heat. Cover the skillet, keeping the spinach warm.

Meanwhile, add about 1 inch of water to a medium saucepan, heating it up on medium heat until it begins to boil. Once it starts boiling, add the salt and vinegar, turning the heat down to low. Break an egg into a small cup, then gently place the egg in the hot water. Do the same thing with each egg. Cover the pan, allowing the water to simmer. Cooking for about 3-5 minutes, shaking from a couple times. Yolks should start thickening and whites should be set when the eggs are done.

One four warmed plates, place half of an English muffin. Place about ¼ of the spinach mixture over the muffin. With a slotted spoon, remove poached eggs, draining them and placing on top of the spinach. Add a tablespoon of the poaching water to the leftover yogurt mixture, stirring it until smooth. Spread the yogurt mixture over eggs. Top with a bit of freshly ground pepper and serve right away. Makes four servings.

Pumpkin Pie Flavored Oatmeal Breakfast Recipe

This is a delicious belly fat buster that tastes amazing. You get the wonderful taste of pumpkin pie while blasting away belly fat. You'll also find that this oatmeal recipe is very filling, helping you avoid cravings throughout your day. Serve up this oatmeal with about a cup of skim milk. This only makes a single serving, so you may want to double or quadruple the recipe if you need to make more.

What You'll Need:

1/3 cup of quick cooking oats
1 teaspoons of brown sugar
1 cup of water
¼ cup of canned pure pumpkin (not pumpkin pie filling)
Pinch of ground cloves
Pinch of nutmeg
Pinch of salt
¼ teaspoon of ground cinnamon
2 tablespoons of pecans, chopped and toasted

How to Make It:

Heat up the water in a medium saucepan. Heat until water is boiling. After water comes to a boil, add the quick oats and the salt to the pan. Allow to cook for about 90 seconds. In a small bowl, combine the pumpkin, brown sugar, cloves, nutmeg, cinnamon and pecans. Reduce the heat of the oatmeal, once on low, stir the pumpkin pecan mixture into the oatmeal. Serve with skim milk. Makes a single serving.

Delicious French Toast with Chocolate Breakfast Recipe

If you have a bit of extra time on the weekend, this recipe is sure to be a hit with the family while going along with your belly fat diet. The great thing about this wonderful French toast recipe is that it offers plenty of fiber and protein for breakfast, which helps to keep you feeling full. Add fruit on the side for a well-rounded breakfast that you're sure to enjoy. After all, it's always nice to start the day with a bit of chocolate.

What You'll Need:

3 ounces of low fat cream cheese, softened
6 ounces of Italian bread, cut into 8 slices about a half inch thick
2 large egg whites
2 large eggs
4 ounces of semi-sweet chocolate, chopped finely
1 tablespoon of margarine, trans fat free
1 tablespoon of sugar
1 teaspoon of vanilla
1 teaspoon of orange zest, freshly grated
2 cups of fresh strawberries, sliced

How to Make It:

In a little bowl, combine the cream cheese and the chocolate together. In another bowl, combine the orange zest, sugar and strawberry slices.

On four slices of the Italian bread, spread a quarter of the cream cheese and chocolate mixture. Top each slice with another slice of bread, pressing slices together lightly.

In a medium sized bowl, combine the vanilla, egg whites and eggs. Whip lightly. Dip each side of the bread into the egg mixture, then setting the sandwich on a platter.

Place margarine in a large skillet, heating it on medium heat. When margarine is completely melted, place sandwiches into the skillet, cooking for about four minutes on each side. French toast should be cooked through and golden brown. Divide the fresh toast among four plates, topping the fresh toast with the strawberry mixture. Serve while hot. Makes four servings.

Belly Melt Huevos Ranchero's Breakfast Recipe

When you try this delicious breakfast recipe, you'll be surprised at all the flavor. It includes plenty of veggies and wonderful herbs add tons of flavor. The eggs give you plenty of protein, while you get your monounsaturated fats from the avocado that is included. If you like a little more kick when you eat your eggs, try adding just a bit of hot pepper sauce to the eggs when you eat them.

What You'll Need:

4 scallions, thinly sliced

1 teaspoon of ground cumin

2 cloves of garlic, minced

4 tablespoons of salsa

1 cup of avocado, sliced

½ cup of chicken broth, reduced-sodium

1 can of pink beans, no salt added, drained and rinsed

1 red bell pepper, sliced into thin strips

4 tablespoons of Greek yogurt, fat free

4 eggs

8 six-inch corn tortillas, toasted

How to Make It:

Begin heating a 10-inch skillet on medium heat. Place cumin in the pan, allowing to cook until it becomes fragrant. Only cook for about 30 seconds, stirring from time to time. Place the garlic, bell pepper, beans, broth and scallions in the skillet with the cumin. Bring the mixture to a boil, then reduce heat, allowing the mixture to simmer. Simmer for about eight minutes, ensuring that the vegetables become very tender and most of the chicken broth evaporates. Use a spoon to smash up the beans, making a thick, lumpy mixture.

With the back of a wooden spoon, make four different indentations in the mixture. Break an egg into a cup, pouring carefully into one of the indentations. Do the same thing with the rest of the eggs. Cover the skillet and allow eggs to cook for 8-10 minutes, ensuring that eggs are done to your taste.

Separate the mixture into four equal parts, ensuring each part has one egg. Place on four plates. Place slices of avocado around the beans. Use the salsa and yogurt to top the dish. Serve up with the toasted tortillas while hot. Makes four servings.

Belly Filling Parfait with Granola Breakfast Recipe

Not only is this parfait a delicious treat, but it is good for you to. You can make it in no time, which makes it great for busy mornings. It also looks elegant, which means you can serve this healthy breakfast up to guests and they'll never know how healthy it really is for them.

What You'll Need:

1 cup of raspberries
1 ½ cups of Granola
1 large banana, sliced
1 small 5.3 ounce container of Greek yogurt, fat free

How to Make It:

Place a small amount of granola in the bottom of a tall glass or parfait cup. Top with granola. Add fruit on top of granola. Repeat layers until the glass is full. Do the same thing in the second glass. Makes two servings, but it's easy to double the recipe to make more.

Decadent Walnut Banana Pancakes Breakfast Recipe

These pancakes are sensational and they'll help you work on gaining a flat belly too. You get a nice combination of crunchy and sweet with the walnuts and honey included in the recipe. The walnuts also add healthy, belly blasting fats to the recipe as well. This recipe includes plenty of fiber too, which means you'll stay feeling full longer. Serve with berries on the side for the perfect breakfast.

What You'll Need:

¼ cup of water

1 tablespoon of canola oil

½ cup of fresh raspberries

1 1/3 pancake mix, trans fat free

1 egg

1 teaspoon of vanilla

1 cup of buttermilk, low fat

¼ teaspoon of ground cinnamon

1 large banana, cut into very thin slices

1/3 cup of honey

1 tablespoon of water

½ cup of chopped walnuts

How to Make It:

In a large mixing bowl, combine the cinnamon and pancake mix. In a smaller bowl, combine the vanilla, egg, oil, buttermilk and water. Whisk the wet ingredients into the dry ingredients, stirring well until you have a smooth mixture. Fold the slices of banana into the pancake batter, setting to the side.

In a small bowl, combine the water, honey and walnuts.

Take a large nonstick skillet, coating it well with cooking spray. Place on medium heat and warm. Once the skillet is hot, begin adding batter by the ¼ cupful, cooking in batches. Pancakes should cook for about 2 minutes on each side, or until they become browned lightly.

Serve up pancakes, dividing among four separate plates. While hot, top with the walnut and honey mixture. Serve the raspberries on the side. Makes four servings.

Pecan and Cranberry Scones Breakfast Recipe

When you want a nice treat for breakfast, these scones are the perfect option. You can easily make a nice batch of the scones at the beginning of the week, storing them in the freezer so you can enjoy them all week. In fact, they are great if you need to grab your breakfast when you're headed out the door. The pecans add the monounsaturated fat to the recipe, helping it blast away your belly fat while enjoying a delicious breakfast.

What You'll Need:

1 ¼ cup of vanilla yogurt, low fat

1 cup of chopped pecans

2/3 cup of sweetened, dried cranberries

2 tablespoons of canola oil

2 cups of whole wheat pastry flour

½ teaspoon of baking soda

1 teaspoon of orange zest, freshly grated

½ teaspoon of salt

2 teaspoons of baking powder

How to Make It:

Preheat oven to 400F.

Coat a 9-inch round baking dish with some nonstick cooking spray.

In a large mixing bowl, mix together the baking powder, salt, baking soda, pecans and flour. In a smaller bowl, combine the orange zest, oil and yogurt. In the middle of the flour mixture, create a well, pouring the yogurt mixture into the well, as well as the cranberries. Stir the mixture until ingredients are blended.

Press the batter into the pan that has been prepared with cooking spray. Use a knife to score the dough, making eight triangles. Bake the scones for about 20-25 minutes. To check for doneness, insert a toothpick into the center. It should come out clean if the scones are done. Makes eight servings.

Nut and Fruit Oatmeal Breakfast Recipe

You probably already know how great oatmeal is for your heart. However, you may be unaware of how great it is for flattening your belly. This oatmeal recipe combines various nuts and fruits, adding plenty of flavor and great healthy fats that work to help you slim down that belly. You'll love the flavor of this oatmeal and you'll be surprised to find that it keeps you feeling full until lunch, so you may not even need a midmorning snack anymore.

What You'll Need:

½ cup of sweetened, dried cranberries
1 ¼ cup of rolled, old-fashioned oats
¼ cup of golden raisins
1 Granny Smith apple
1 cup of water
½ cup of walnuts, chopped
2 ½ cups of skim milk, divided

How to Make It:

Begin by washing the apple. Once washed, core the apple and then cut apple into ¼-inch chunks.

In a large saucepan, add 1 ½ cup of milk and the cup of water, bringing it to a boil with high heat. Stir in the oats, adding a pinch of salt if you desire. Heat should be reduced to low, allowing the oats to simmer for 3-4 minutes as the oats soften. Stir regularly.

Add the chopped apple to the oats. Cover the pan, allowing the oatmeal to simmer for about 3-4 more minutes. Oats should be slightly crisp, yet tender. Add raisins and cranberries. Remove the oatmeal from the heat, covering again and allowing it to stand for 1-2 minutes or until completely softened.

Scoop out oatmeal, dividing it up among four medium size bowls. Top each bowl of oatmeal with a ½ teaspoon of brown sugar and two tablespoons of the chopped walnuts. Add ¼ cup of the leftover skim milk to each bowl. Serve immediately. Makes four servings.

Chapter 5: Great Lunch Recipes to Help You Lose Belly Fat

It's important to eat a good lunch, since it will keep you from eating unhealthy snacks between lunch and dinner. Salads are always a great option for lunch and you'll find plenty of great salad recipes that fit in with your belly fat diet. Enjoy many tasty flavors while working to eliminate more belly fat. Try mixing up these recipes so you don't end up eating a salad every day, ensuring you don't get bored of salads.

Easy Turkey Pita with Side Salad Lunch Recipe

When you need a quick and easy lunch, this recipe is the perfect choice. The turkey offers plenty of great lean protein, plus, the veggies are great for helping you get that flat belly you desire. The olive oil in the side salad is a healthy, fat fighting, monounsaturated fat and the unique extras like the hearts of palm make sure you won't be bored with this salad.

What You'll Need:

Pita

1/8 cup of sprouts
¼ cup of baby spinach
4 ounces of turkey
1 whole wheat pita, small
4 small slices of tomato
1 teaspoon of Dijon mustard

Side Salad

½ cup of hearts of palm
1 cup of romaine lettuce, chopped
½ cup of red pepper, chopped
1 teaspoon of olive oil

½ cup of cucumber, chopped

How to Make It:

Cut the whole wheat pita in half. Spread insides of the pita with the mustard. Add slices of turkey to each half of the pita. Top with the sprouts, tomato slices and spinach.

Wash all the vegetables for the salad. Chop the romaine, peppers, cucumbers and cut up the hearts of palm into smaller pieces if needed. Toss all salad ingredients together. Drizzle the salad with the olive oil.

Makes a single serving.

Shrimp, Barley and Baby Green Salad Lunch Recipe

The curry powder and turmeric add a delicious flavor to this recipe, making it a salad that won't make you bored. The shrimp adds plenty of healthy protein to the salad without adding a lot of calories. The wide variety of vegetables makes sure you get plenty of crunch when you eat this salad, while you'll get some healthy fat from the pumpkin seeds added to the mix.

What You'll Need:

1 cup of barley

¼ cup of fresh basil, chopped

1 tablespoons of vegetable oil

3 cups of water

1 pound of shrimp, peeled, deveined and cooked

½ cup of cucumber, peeled and chopped

1 teaspoon of curry powder

1 tablespoons of lime juice, freshly squeezed

1 clove of garlic, minced

¾ cup of pumpkin seeds, toasted

1 ½ cups of tomatoes, diced and seeded

½ teaspoon of turmeric

2 teaspoons of jalapeno chili pepper, seeded and finely chopped

12 cups of baby greens

½ cup of green bell pepper, chopped

¼ teaspoon of salt

¼ cup of lemon juice

How to Make It:

Bring the water, turmeric and curry to a boil in a large saucepan. Once water is boiling, add the barley to the water. Cover the pan, reducing the heat and allowing to simmer. Allow barley to cook for approximately 40-45 minutes, until the barley becomes tender and the water has been absorbed. Remove barley from the heat.

While barley is cooking, whisk the oil, garlic, lime juice, lemon juice, salt and chili pepper together. Add the cucumber, tomatoes, shrimp, barley and bell pepper to the dressing mixture. Toss well to coat evenly.

On six plates, place two cups of the baby greens on each plate. Divide up the shrimp salad, adding salad on top of the bed of greens. Top with the pumpkin seeds and basil. Makes six servings.

Rainbow Veggie, Soba Noodle and Chicken Salad Lunch Recipe

The soba noodles, which can be substituted with whole wheat spaghetti, adds a nice amount of fiber to this salad. You'll get plenty of veggies from the peppers, snow peas and carrots. The avocado offers the monounsaturated fats you need in this meal. The soy sauce, pepper flakes, peanut oil and ginger really add a nice flavor to this salad. The bit of honey keeps the pucker factor under control.

What You'll Need:

2 tablespoons of lime juice, freshly squeezed
2 red bell peppers, seeded and sliced thinly
1 tablespoon of fresh ginger, grated
¼ cup of fresh cilantro, chopped coarsely
8 ounces of dry soba noodles or the same amount of whole wheat spaghetti
¼ teaspoon of red pepper flakes
2 cups of fresh snow peas, julienned
1 ½ cups of avocado, diced
2 tablespoons of honey
2 tablespoons of soy sauce, reduced sodium
2 tablespoons of peanut oil
1 cup of carrots, grated

2 cups of cooked chicken, shredded
2 tablespoons of rice wine vinegar

How to Make It:

Cook the soba noodles or spaghetti noodles according to the directions on the package. Once noodles are done cooking, drain well and then rinse with some cold water to ensure they stop cooking. Set noodles to the side.

Whisk the lime juice, ginger, soy sauce, vinegar, pepper flakes and honey together in a large bowl. Add the peanut oil in a steady stream while whisking the mixture. After dressing is well mixed, fold the bell peppers, avocado, noodles, cilantro, snow peas, carrots and chicken into the dressing. Serve immediately or chill and serve later. Makes six servings.

Mediterranean Style Wraps Lunch Recipe

The olive tapenade that is used in these wraps is an excellent source of monounsaturated fats, boosting the belly busting power of these tasty wraps. The chickpeas offer great protein to the wraps, while you'll get plenty of crunch from the peppers, onions and greens. The lemon juice and goat cheese makes these wraps full of incredible flavor. Make them the night before and take them to work for a healthy lunch that will keep you from eating out and ruining your belly fat diet.

What You'll Need:

4 cups of salad greens of choice

½ of a small red onion, sliced thinly

½ cup of canned chickpeas, no salt added, drained and rinsed

½ cup of green olive tapenade

2 ounces of goat cheese, crumbled

2 tablespoons of lemon juice, freshly squeezed

½ cup of jarred roasted red peppers, drained, sliced and dried

4 whole wheat tortillas or wraps (8-inches)

½ cup of seedless cucumber, sliced thinly

How to Make It:

In a large bowl, mix the lemon juice and green olive tapenade together with a fork. Add the peppers, onion, cucumber, greens and chickpeas to the mix, tossing to ensure they are well mixed. Add the goat cheese to the bowl, tossing gently to avoid breaking up the cheese further.

Warm the tortillas or wraps according to the directions on the package. Place a quarter of the mixture on the bottom of one of the wraps, rolling up securely. Cut the wrap in half at an angle, using a toothpick to keep the wraps together. Do the same thing with each of the wraps. Makes four servings.

Low Sugar Strawberry and Peanut Butter Wraps Lunch Recipe

Peanut butter and jelly is a timeless classic that is a favorite among kids and adults alike. This recipe brings you all the flavor that comes with a peanut butter and jelly sandwich. However, since it uses fruit instead of jelly, you don't have to worry about a meal that includes a lot of unneeded sugar. Also, the wraps add plenty of fiber to the meal, helping you stay full throughout the afternoon. Make these wraps to take to work and make a few extras for the kids as well. Everyone is sure to enjoy these healthy wraps that also help to shrink your belly.

What You'll Need:

1 cup of strawberries, sliced
2 8-inch whole wheat tortillas
4 tablespoons of natural crunchy peanut butter, preferably unsalted

How to Make It:

Place the tortillas on a work area. Spread each tortilla with half of the peanut butter, spreading carefully to avoid tearing the tortilla with the nuts in the peanut butter. Cover each tortilla with half of the strawberry slices. Roll each tortilla up. Slice diagonally into three sections. Makes two servings.

Easy Whole Wheat Muffin Pizzas Lunch Recipe

Whole wheat English muffins are much better for you than white ones, offering more fiber and a low calorie count. If you enjoy pizza, this is a great way to enjoy some of the wonderful flavors of pizza while sticking to your belly fat diet. You'll get delicious cheeses, great flavor from the basil and plenty of belly fat fighting healthy fats from the black tapenade used on the pizzas. They are easy to make and ready in no time, meaning you'll have a nice weekend lunch ready in a flash.

What You'll Need:

1 tomato, cut up into eight slices
4 teaspoons of Parmesan cheese, grated
½ cup of black tapenade
8 basil leaves, fresh
1 cup of reduced fat mozzarella cheese, shredded
4 whole wheat English muffins, split in half

How to Make It:

Preheat oven to 400F.

After splitting the English muffins, toast them. Once toasted, each muffin half should be spread with about a tablespoon of the black tapenade. 1 tomato slice should go on each muffin half. Top the tomatoes with a ½ teaspoon of Parmesan cheese and about 2 tablespoons of the mozzarella.

Place each English muffin half on a baking sheet. Place pizzas in the oven, allowing to take for 6-8 minutes, ensuring that the cheese is well melted. Remove from the oven, topping with a leaf of basil before serving. Serve right away. Makes four servings. You can also make extras and store them in the fridge for a couple days. They make a great snack.

Walnut and Radish Spinach Salad Lunch Recipe

While the walnuts and olive oil add the important monounsaturated fats to this recipe, the baby spinach and radishes offer plenty of important nutrients for the body. The lemon juice, white wine vinegar and black pepper produce plenty of great flavor. Not only does this salad make a wonderful lunch recipe, but it's a nice side dish that can be served up with dinner as well.

What You'll Need:

4 medium sized radishes, sliced thinly
1 tablespoon of lemon juice, freshly squeezed
¼ cup of extra virgin olive oil
½ cup of walnuts, halved
2 teaspoons of white wine vinegar
5 ounces of baby spinach
Black pepper, freshly ground, to taste
Salt, to taste

How to Make It:

Whisk the vinegar and lemon juice together in a large bowl. Add pepper and salt to taste. Slowly pour in the olive oil, whisking continually.

Right before serving, toss the radishes and spinach with the dressing, coating greens completely. Divide up the salad among four different salad plates. Top the salad with walnuts. Serve right away. Makes four servings.

Chapter 6: Flat Belly Diet Dinner Recipes

Eating a good dinner will help you avoid those late night snack cravings, which can quickly sabotage your belly fat diet. All of these recipes include some form of monounsaturated fat, which helps to blast away that belly fat that you are working so hard to lose. You'll find great fish recipes, meatless recipes and more. Even if you need a dinner in a hurry, you'll find easy, fast recipes that allow you to eat a healthy dinner, even on your busiest days.

Smoked Salmon Frittata Dinner Recipe

It's always nice to have a breakfast style recipe for dinner. This dinner recipe makes use of eggs and salmon, ensuring you get plenty of protein. The salmon is full of healthy Omega-3s, which are important if you want to enjoy a flatter belly. The combination of protein and healthy fats help ensure you won't be reaching for a late night snack later in the evening.

What You'll Need:

4 eggs
6 egg whites
2 ounces of smoked salmon, thinly sliced and cut into pieces (about ½-inch wide)
6 scallions, trimmed and chopped coarsely
¼ cup of cold water
¾ cup of black olive tapenade
½ teaspoon of salt
1 ½ teaspoons of fresh tarragon, chopped
2 teaspoons of extra virgin olive oil
Black pepper, freshly ground

How to Make It:

Preheat oven to 350F.

On medium heat, heat up an 8-inch skillet that is ovenproof, heating on medium for about a minute. Place olive oil in the skillet, adding scallions to the oil. Sauté the scallions until they are soft, stirring regularly.

Whisk the tarragon, salt, egg whites, water and eggs together in a medium sized bowl. Add black pepper to taste. Pour the egg mixture into the skillet, topping with the pieces of salmon. Allow to cook for about two minutes, stirring from time to time, allowing eggs to set partially.

Place the skillet with the egg mixture into the oven, allowing to cook for 6-8 minutes. Eggs should be puffed, firm and golden brown on top. Remove the skillet from the oven. Release the frittata from the skillet with a spatula. Slide carefully onto a serving platter that has been warmed.

On six plates, spread about two tablespoons of the black olive tapenade. Top the tapenade with a slice of frittata. Eat immediately while hot. Makes six servings.

Chicken Breast with Almond Crust Dinner Recipe

Chicken packs a powerful protein punch, but it's lower in fat than certain other meats, as long as you don't use the skin. This recipe calls for skinless and boneless chicken breasts, so you don't have to worry about removing the skin. The almond crust makes the chicken something special and also keeps the inside from drying out while you cook it. Serve up with some tomatoes and cottage cheese on the side for a wonderful meal that will keep you feeling satisfied. Keep in mind, this recipe is only for a single serving, so if you're feeling a family or guests, you may need to make extra to fit your needs.

What You'll Need:

1 tablespoon of cornstarch
2 tablespoons of almonds, chopped finely
¼ cup of egg substitute, fat free
5 ounces of skinless, boneless chicken breast

How to Make It:

Sprinkle chicken breasts generously with cornstarch on both sides. After nicely coated with the cornstarch, dip the chicken breast into the egg substitute, ensuring it's well coated. After coated with the egg substitute, sprinkle the chopped almonds over the chicken on both sides.

Spray nonstick cooking spray on a nonstick skillet, heating it up on medium. Place chicken breast in the skilled, cooking for about five minutes per side until done. The thickest part of the chicken breast should reach 165 degrees F to make it safe to consume. Makes a single serving.

Easy Belly Busting Slow Cooker Chili Dinner Recipe

This chili recipe is so easy to make. Since you can put it in the slow cooker, it makes dinner so easy for busy individuals that want a meal that is ready to eat for dinner. With olive oil and avocados, you're getting the fat busting monounsaturated fats that you need. The chili beans add extra protein to the chili and instead of meat, soy crumbles are used, allowing you to enjoy a nice, meat-free dish from time to time.

What You'll Need:

1 can of chili beans (14 oz.), drained and rinsed
1 tablespoon of extra virgin olive oil
1 green bell pepper, seeded and then diced
Chili powder to taste
1 cup of avocado, chopped
1 can of whole tomatoes, salt free (28 oz.)
1 tablespoon of onion, minced
12 ounces of soy crumbles, fat free

How to Make It:

Combine the soy crumbles, onion, oil, chili powder, pepper, tomatoes and beans in a four quart slow cooker.

Cover the slow cooker, cooking on low for 8-10 hours or on high for 4-6 hours. Chili should be well thickened by the time it's done cooking. Scoop chili into four bowls. Top with avocado pieces and serve hot. Makes four servings.

Snow Peas and Steamed Gingered Salmon Dinner Recipe

Salmon is a great protein choice to eat while you are trying to slim down that belly. Not only does it provide a low calorie form of protein, but it also includes healthy fats that help to eliminate that belly fat. The sesame oil, lime juice, ginger, garlic and soy sauce all make a delicious glaze that provides the great flavor for this steamed salmon. Chopped avocado adds even more healthy fats to the meal and the snow peas round it out to be an easy meal that won't take long to fix for dinner.

What You'll Need:

1 clove of garlic, minced

1 cup of avocado, chopped

1 teaspoon of fresh ginger, grated

2 scallions, sliced thinly

1 tablespoon of lime juice, freshly squeezed

1 pound of trimmed snow peas

1 teaspoon of toasted sesame oil

2 teaspoons of soy sauce, reduced sodium

4 salmon fillets, skinless and about 1.5 inches thick

How to Make It:

Rub the garlic and ginger on the salmon fillets. Use nonstick cooking spray to coat a steaming basket. Place the salmon fillets into the basket. Bring about two inches of water to boiling in a large saucepan. Add the steamer basket to the pan, covering and allowing the salmon to steam for about 7-9 minutes.

While the salmon is steaming, whisk the soy sauce, scallions, oil and lime juice together in a small bowl, setting to the side for later.

Once the salmon has been steaming for 7-9 minutes, add the snow peas on top of the salmon in the steamer basket. Allow the peas and salmon to steam for another 4-5 minutes, making sure that salmon is well cooked and the peas are tender yet crispy.

On four plates, arrange snow peas to make a bed for the salmon. Top the snow peas with the salmon. Top each salmon fillet with some of the avocado pieces. Drizzle with the soy sauce mixture. Serve right away while hot. Makes four servings.

Chicken Roulade Stuffed with Spinach Dinner Recipe

Not only does this delicious chicken recipe taste amazing, but it looks great served up on dinner plates as well. It's easy enough to make for a family dinner at home. However, it's elegant enough to make for guests as well. Enjoy plenty of flavor with the red pepper flakes and the sun dried tomatoes. The spinach adds plenty of nutrition to this healthy dish as well.

What You'll Need:

2 teaspoons of olive oil
½ cup of dry white wine or chicken broth
¼ cup of onion, finely chopped
¼ cup of Parmesan cheese, grated
1 10oz package of frozen chopped spinach
1/3 teaspoon of red pepper flakes
2 tablespoons of dry packed sun dried tomatoes, chopped
1 clove of garlic, grated or crushed
4 chicken breast halves, carefully trimmed and pounded into very thin cutlets

How to Make It:

Make the frozen spinach according to the directions on the package. Once cooked, place spinach in a strainer, using a spoon to help press out the extra liquid. You should have about ½ cup of spinach left.

While spinach is cooking, place a teaspoon of the olive oil in a nonstick skillet, heating on medium heat. Add the garlic, onion, 1 tablespoon of water and the red pepper flakes to the skillet. Allow to cook until onion begins to sizzle. Reduce heat to low, covering and allowing to cook until the onion is softened, which should take about 2-4 minutes. Stir once while cooking.

When spinach is ready, stir the spinach, cheese and onion mixture together in a little bowl. Keep the skillet to the side to use later.

On the smooth side of the chicken cutlets, sprinkle with the tomatoes. Divide the spinach mixture, spreading it evenly on each cutlet. Leave about an inch at the narrow end without the spread. Roll up the chicken cutlets loosely, using a wooden toothpick to secure it.

Add the rest of the olive oil to the previously used skilled. Heat oil on medium heat, adding the chicken to the skillet, browning chicken on every side for about 10 minutes. Add the dry white wine to the skillet, covering the skillet and allowing the chicken to cook on low for another 7-8 minutes. Uncover the pan, moving chicken to a warm serving dish. Use foil to cover the chicken, keeping it warm until serving.

Bring the leftover juices in the skillet to a boil until you have a nice glaze. This should take approximately 4-5 minutes. Slice the chicken roulades diagonally into pieces about an inch thick. Drizzle with the glaze and then serve while warm. Makes four servings.

Easy Whole Wheat Veggie Pizza Recipe

As you work hard to lose belly fat, you still do not want to give up some of your favorite foods. The good news is that you can still enjoy having pizza while you are on the flat belly diet. This recipe makes use of many great veggies that will fill you up while allowing you to enjoy some pizza. The mixture of mozzarella cheese, Parmesan cheese, basil, mushrooms, peppers and pesto will provide you with plenty of great flavor as you enjoy this delicious pizza dish.

What You'll Need:

½ cup of finely sliced red onion

¾ cup of cherry tomatoes, quartered

¼ cup of sun-dried tomato pesto

2 tablespoons of Parmesan cheese, grated

2 teaspoons of olive oil

1 cup of button mushrooms, sliced

1 cup of sliced zucchini

½ cup of basil leaves, thinly sliced

1 cup of yellow or orange bell peppers, sliced thinly

1 whole wheat pizza crust, thin

How to Make It:

Begin by preheating the oven to 425F.

Work the whole wheat pizza crust out on the pizza pan, ensuring the entire pan is covered with the crust. Take the pesto and spread it out evenly over the crust. Place the peppers, onion, mushrooms and zucchini in a bowl. Pour in the olive oil. Toss the vegetables in the olive oil until they are coated.

Place veggies in a skillet heated over medium heat. Saute the vegetables for 5-8 minutes or until the veggies have turned soft and the liquid from the veggies has evaporated.

Sprinkle the cheeses over the crust, making sure the crust is covered evenly. Take the sautéed veggies and add them to the pizza crust on top of the cheese. Top the pizza with the tomato pieces.

Place the pizza in the oven, allowing to bake for 18-20 minutes. The crust should be baked throughout and should be crisped slightly on the bottom. Remove from the oven. While hot, sprinkle the pizza with the sliced basil leaves. Allow to stand for 5 minutes. Cut the pizza into quarters and then serve. Makes four servings.

Roasted Pepper and Portobello Mushroom Burgers Recipe

If you find yourself craving the delicious flavor of a burger while you are following the flat belly diet, you will definitely love this tasty recipe. You do not have to worry about the calories and fat that comes with beef, since no meat is used within this recipe. Portobello mushroom caps make up the burger part of the recipes and these mushrooms are full of rich, delicious flavor that will let you enjoy the flavor of a burger without all the fat and calories. The addition of roasted bell peppers and pesto really amp up the flavor, making this a burger that will make your taste buds sing while you enjoy working on a flatter belly.

What You'll Need:

2 roasted red bell pepper halves, jarred
4 leaves of frisee lettuce, or other lettuce you have on hand
4 small to medium Portobello mushroom caps, about 8 ounces
2 tablespoons of pesto, prepared
4 teaspoons of balsamic vinegar
2 whole wheat hamburger buns

How to Make It:

Over medium heat, preheat a large grill pan.

Place the Portobello mushroom caps on the grill pan, grilling them for four minutes on each side. While mushroom caps are cooking, continue to brush with the balsamic vinegar. When mushrooms are nearly done, warm the buns and the bell pepper halves on the grill pan too.

Spread half of the pesto on each of the hamburger buns. On the bottom of each bun, place 1 of the red pepper slices and two mushroom caps. Top with 2 pieces of the lettuce. If desired, add just a little bit more vinegar. Top with the top of the bun. Enjoy immediately. Makes two servings.

Pepper Steak Tacos Dinner Recipe

Eating lean protein and whole grains can help you enjoy flatter abs and this delicious recipe includes some of the best belly slimming ingredients to make a delicious dinner. The flank steak used within the recipe offers a lot of lean protein. You will get plenty of veggies in this dish as well, including bell peppers, corn, avocado, jalapenos and more. Enjoy making this recipe up for a nice dinner. You may even want to make some extras so you can take some to work for a nice, healthy lunch.

What You'll Need:

3 teaspoons of olive oil

½ cup of frozen or fresh corn kernels

¼ cup of Monterey Jack cheese, low fat, grated

2 cloves of garlic, crushed

1 lime, juiced + lime wedges when serving the dish

½ teaspoon of mild chili powder

¼ cup of salsa Verde

3 bell peppers, thinly sliced (1 orange, 1 red and 1 yellow)

1 teaspoon of kosher salt

½ red onion, thinly sliced

½ avocado, sliced

2 tablespoons of pickled jalapenos, sliced

1 pound of flank steak
Light sour cream to taste

How to Make It:

Mix together the lime juice, crushed garlic, chili powder and salt in a sealable plastic bag. Add the flank steak to the bag, shaking up so the marinade coats the steak. Place the marinating steak into the refrigerator for about 20-30 minutes, minimum.

While the steak is marinating, place a cast iron skillet on medium high heat until well heated. Add two teaspoons of the olive oil to the skillet. Place the bell peppers and red onion in the skillet, allowing to cook for about five minutes, tossing and stirring while cooking. Place the corn kernels in the skillet, continuing to cook the vegetables for about 3-4 more minutes or until the peppers become soft and slightly charred. When veggies are done cooking, place them in a medium bowl and place in the microwave to keep warm.

Use a paper towel to wipe out the skillet. Heat the skillet for a minute and then add in the leftover teaspoon of the olive oil. Take steak out of the marinade, using paper towels to pat it dry. Place the steak in the pan and cook over medium high heat for four minutes on each side.

Once the steak is done cooking, remove it from the pan and place on a cutting board. Allow the steak to rest for 5-7 minutes.

Use a sharp knife to slice the flank steak, cutting across the grain. Arrange the steak on a large platter with lime wedges and peppers. Warm tortillas and then begin making tacos. Place steak and peppers in the tortillas, adding avocado, cheese, jalapenos, salsa and the sour cream. Enjoy. Makes four servings.

Belly Flattening Broccoli Rabe Sausage Penne Recipe

Whole wheat pasta is a great addition to your belly fat diet. It fills you up but it does not spike blood sugar like white pasta does. Instead of using traditional, high fat sausages, this recipe uses turkey sausages, which offer a lot of protein without all the fat usually found in sausage. This recipe gets plenty of flavor from the crushed red pepper flakes, ricotta cheese and the Parmesan cheese. The great thing about this recipe is that you can have it ready in under a half hour, making it a quick, easy dinner to use during the week when you are really busy.

What You'll Need:

½ red onion, sliced thinly
12 ounces of whole wheat penne pasta
2 tablespoons of tomato paste
1 clove of garlic, thinly sliced
2 tablespoons of Parmesan, grated
1 medium bunch of broccoli rabe
2 Italian turkey sausages with the casings removed
¼ cup of ricotta cheese, part skim
Pinch of crushed red pepper flakes
1 tablespoon of extra virgin olive oil

How to Make It:

Fill a large pot with water, adding a bit of salt. Bring the water to a boil. Once boiling, add the broccoli rabe to the water, allowing it to cook for about 3-5 minutes. Remove broccoli rabe from the boiling water, placing it in a colander to drain and cool. Once you can handle it, chop it up into bite-size chunks.

Bring the same pot of water back to boiling. Place the whole wheat penne in the boiling water. Cook until it is al dente. Set aside ½ cup of the pasta water and then drain the penne pasta.

While the penne is cooking, place a large skillet over medium heat. Add the olive oil and allow it to heat up. Add the garlic, onion, red pepper flakes and sausages to the hot olive oil. Use a wooden spoon to break up the sausages. Cook the mixture until the sausages are well browned, which will take about eight minutes. Then, place the broccoli rabe into the pan with the sausage mixture, continuing to cook until the rabe becomes tender, about 2-3 more minutes.

Turn the heat under the skillet down to low. Place the drained pasta in the skillet with the sausage mixture.

Toss well to make sure all the ingredients are combined. If the mixture seems a bit dry, add a small amount of the reserved pasta water to the pan. Stir the Parmesan and ricotta cheeses into the pan, removing the pan from the heat and tossing again. Serve the pasta dish right away. Makes six servings.

Chapter 7: Belly Flattening Drink, Snack and Dessert Recipes

Ricotta and Citrus Cannoli Dessert Recipe

Just because you're following a belly fat diet doesn't mean that you have to skip out on a tasty dessert. This dessert will go well with your diet, helping you to achieve the flat belly you really want. Of course, you shouldn't overindulge on these delicious delicacies, but it's fine to enjoy one from time to time. It also makes a wonderful, belly friendly dessert to make if you're having guests for dinner. It goes wonderful with a few slices of banana and strawberries on the side.

What You'll Need:

1 tablespoon of orange zest, freshly grated
½ teaspoon of pure vanilla extract
1/3 cup of powdered sugar
3 cups of chocolate chips, semi-sweet, divided
16-ounces of ricotta cheese, fat free

1 teaspoon of lime zest, freshly grated

2 teaspoons of lemon zest, freshly grated

12 cannoli shells, large

How to Make It:

Combine the vanilla, orange zest, lime zest, lemon zest, powdered sugar and ricotta in a medium sized mixing bowl. Use an electric mixer to whip the mixture together until it becomes fluffy and very light. Fold 2 ½ cups of the chocolate chips into the ricotta mixture, saving the last ½ cup of chocolate chips for later.

Take cannoli shells, dividing up the filling evenly among the shells. Use a spoon to get the filling into the shells or you can pipe it in with a plastic bag that has the tip cut off. Melt the rest of the chocolate chips. Drizzle the chocolate on top of every cannoli. Allow chocolate to harden. Place in the refrigerator. Serve cannoli chilled. Makes 12 servings.

Tasty Strawberry Tropical Fruit Smoothie Recipe

Just a taste of this delicious smoothie is like being in paradise. Enjoy sipping on this drink while imagining you are far away on the beach. Not only does this smoothie taste amazing, but it is good for you. It will help you lose weight and flatten that belly, especially since it adds in some flaxseed oil to the mix. When you are craving something a bit sweet, this will help you fix that craving.

What You'll Need:

1 cup of vanilla yogurt, fat free
1 ½ cup of frozen peach slices
½ cup of mango nectar, chilled
1 cup of fresh strawberries, hulled and cut in half
2 tablespoons of flaxseed oil
1 tablespoon of frozen pineapple juice concentrate, thawed slightly

How to Make It:

In a large blender, place the yogurt, frozen peach slices, mango nectar, strawberries and the pineapple juice concentrate. Blend the ingredients until they become smooth and well combined. Once well blended, add the flaxseed oil to the blender, only blending enough to combine thoroughly.

Pour the blender contents into two large glasses. Add a strawberry half to each glass as a garnish. Enjoy the smoothie right away. Makes two servings.

Delicious Apple Yogurt Dessert Recipe

This wonderful apple yogurt dessert recipe allows you to enjoy something sweet without sabotaging your belly fat diet. You will get to enjoy all the flavors found in apple crisp without the high calories and fat that come with that tasty dessert. The addition of Greek yogurt makes sure you get plenty of protein while you enjoy a sweet treat. Make this for dessert after dinner or enjoy it as a sweet snack at any time of day.

What You'll Need:

2 tablespoons of apple sauce
¾ cup of plain Greek yogurt (or vanilla)
1 teaspoon of honey
Pinch of nutmeg
Pinch of cinnamon
1 Granny smith apple, cored, peeled and diced

How to Make It:

In a small bowl, mix together the apple sauce, honey and Greek yogurt. Stir in the diced apple. Top with a pinch of nutmeg and cinnamon. Mix everything together. Eat right away. Makes a single serving. You may want to double or triple the recipe if you want to serve this dish up to the family as a dessert.

Mocha Protein Health Snack Bites Recipe

If you find yourself craving some chocolate, these delicious mocha bits will help you to quash that craving. Not only will you get your chocolate hit, but you will also get some protein when you eat these bites as well. Keep a couple with you during the day for a tasty, protein rich snack that will keep you going and help you reduce other cravings. They are very easy to make and everyone is sure to enjoy them.

What You'll Need:

6 egg whites
1 teaspoon of coffee
¾ cup of oatmeal
2 granny smith apples, diced
¼ teaspoon of baking powder
1 scoop of chocolate protein shake powder
1 drop of vanilla extract
¼ cup of Quaker oats
2 tablespoons of apple sauce
1 teaspoon of honey
½ teaspoon of cinnamon

How to Make It:

Preheat the oven to 350F.

Place the egg whites, coffee, oatmeal, baking powder, protein shake powder, vanilla, Quaker oats, apple sauce, honey and cinnamon in a blender. Blend the ingredients together until you have a thick mixture. Pour the mixture into a large bowl. Add the diced apples to the mixture, using a spoon to mix the apples into the mix.

Spray an 8x8 inch baking dish with cooking spray. Pour the mixture into the baking dish. Place the baking dish in the oven, baking the mixture for about 25-30 minutes. Remove from the oven and allow to cool.

Once the bites have cooled, cut into eight equal pieces. Makes eight servings. Store bites in a container for up to 3 days.

Delicious Peanut Butter Balls Recipe

Not only do these peanut butter balls make a wonderful dessert or snack, but they pack a great protein punch as well, which can help you meet your flat belly goals. They are really easy to make and once you make up the balls, you'll have a quick snack or dessert that you can grab when you have a craving. Since they have a lot of protein, they will help you stay full and enable you to stick with your belly fat diet.

What You'll Need:

1 teaspoon of vanilla extract
1 cup of Stevia, Splenda or another sugar alternative
4 scoops of vanilla or chocolate protein powder
1 cup of peanut butter, sugar free

How to Make It:

Place the vanilla, sugar alternative, protein powder and peanut butter in a medium bowl. Mix the ingredients together until they are well combined. After the ingredients are well mixed, take tablespoon sized portions and roll them into bowls, placing on wax paper. Once all the balls are rolled, place in the refrigerator until the peanut butter balls are set. Store in an airtight container.

Chapter 8: Your 7 Day Belly Fat Diet Meal Plan

Getting started on a new diet is always difficult, especially when you are trying to figure out how to plan meals so you stick with it. To make it easier for you to stay on your belly fat diet, you can follow this 7-day belly fat diet meal plan. It provides great meals for breakfast, lunch and dinner, as well as some great snack ideas. Follow this plan for the first few days to get you started. Once you are used to the diet, you can mix and match recipes within the book as you continue working to lose that belly fat.

Day 1:

Breakfast: Tomato Pesto Eggs Florentine Breakfast Recipe

Lunch: Easy Whole Wheat Muffin Pizzas Lunch Recipe

Dinner: Chicken Breast with Almond Crust Dinner Recipe

Snack: Mocha Protein Health Snack Bites Recipe

Day 2:

Breakfast: Banana Walnut Breakfast Muffin Recipe

Lunch: Mediterranean Style Wraps Lunch Recipe

Dinner: Snow Peas and Steamed Gingered Salmon Dinner Recipe

Snack: Tasty Strawberry Tropical Fruit Smoothie Recipe

Day 3:

Breakfast: Delicious French Toast with Chocolate Breakfast Recipe

Lunch: Walnut and Radish Spinach Salad Lunch Recipe

Dinner: Smoked Salmon Frittata Dinner Recipe

Snack: Delicious Peanut Butter Balls Recipe

Day 4:

Breakfast: Pumpkin Pie Flavored Oatmeal Breakfast Recipe

Lunch: Low Sugar Strawberry and Peanut Butter Wraps Lunch Recipe

Dinner: Easy Belly Busting Slow Cooker Chili Dinner Recipe

Snack:

Day 5:

Breakfast: Belly Filling Parfait with Granola Breakfast Recipe

Lunch: Easy Turkey Pita with Side Salad Lunch Recipe

Dinner: Chicken Roulade Stuffed with Spinach Dinner Recipe

Snack: Ricotta and Citrus Cannoli Dessert Recipe

Day 6:

Breakfast: Belly Melt Huevos Ranchero's Breakfast Recipe

Lunch: Rainbow Veggie, Soba Noodle and Chicken Salad Lunch Recipe

Dinner: Roasted Pepper and Portobello Mushroom Burgers Recipe

Snack: Leftover Delicious Peanut Butter Balls

Day 7:

Breakfast: Pecan and Cranberry Scones Breakfast Recipe

Lunch: Shrimp, Barley and Baby Green Salad Lunch Recipe

Dinner: Easy Whole Wheat Veggie Pizza Recipe

Snack: Delicious Apple Yogurt Dessert Recipe

Lightning Source UK Ltd.
Milton Keynes UK
UKOW06f0019281015

261472UK00001B/35/P